D0216467

Inside Coma

Inside Coma

A New View of Awareness, Healing, and Hope

Pierre Morin, MD, PhD,
and Gary Reiss, LCSW, PhD

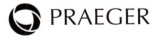 PRAEGER

AN IMPRINT OF ABC-CLIO, LLC
Santa Barbara, California • Denver, Colorado • Oxford, England

Library of Congress Cataloging-in-Publication Data

Morin, Pierre, 1956–
    Inside coma : a new view of awareness, healing, and hope / Pierre Morin and Gary Reiss.
      p. cm.
    Includes bibliographical references and index.
    ISBN 978-0-313-38389-2 (hard copy : alk. paper)—ISBN 978-0-313-38390-8 (ebook)
    1. Coma—Patients—Rehabilitation. I. Reiss, Gary. II. Title.
    [DNLM: 1. Coma—rehabilitation. 2. Psychotherapy—methods. 3. Holistic
Health. WB 182 M858i 2010]
    RB150.C6M67 2010
    616.8'49—dc22   2010007904

ISBN: 978-0-313-38389-2
EISBN: 978-0-313-38390-8

14   13   12   11   10   1   2   3   4   5

This book is also available on the World Wide Web as an eBook.
Visit www.abc-clio.com for details.

Praeger
An Imprint of ABC-CLIO, LLC

ABC-CLIO, LLC
130 Cremona Drive, P.O. Box 1911
Santa Barbara, California 93116-1911

This book is printed on acid-free paper ∞

Manufactured in the United States of America

Contents

vi   **Contents**

Introduction

What is coma?

What is a vegetative state?

What are the possibilities for consciousness in coma?

What makes a life worth living?

In the wake of Terri Schiavo's publicly debated fate and the awakenings of patients from their minimally conscious states after as much as 20 years of silence, we are finally waking up to these questions. Traumatic brain injury affects more Americans each year than breast cancer, multiple sclerosis, HIV/AIDS, and spinal cord injury combined.[1] Many of them will spend time in remote states of consciousness and coma without being able to communicate with the outer world. The fascination with people in comas is everywhere, on magazine covers featuring people like Terri Schiavo, Terry Wallis, and Sarah Scantlin; on *Coma*, Liz Garbus's HBO special that is giving voice to people who have experienced brain injury, in the newspapers and on radio shows; and in movies such as *The Only Thrill*, *Nova*, *Just Like Heaven*, and *The Diving Bell and the Butterfly*. New exciting scientific discoveries are now beginning to validate what we have been noticing and teaching about for years, which is that coma patients' awareness is much more detailed and complex than previously thought, and so are their chances of significant recovery.

A woman who was thought to have no consciousness is able to play tennis in her mind in a way that was measurable.[2] Another person who was given no chance of recovery suddenly speaks after 20 years. People in comas fill hospital beds worldwide, and yet we rarely hear their stories unless it is the occasional amazing person who suddenly wakes up after many years. In many ways, today's medicine ignores them and denies them any living experience. Over many years of working with coma patients, we have found that this hopelessness is unjustified.

In our practical experience, up to a third of the clients we work with who are given no hope of recovery actually do make significant progress, often returning to the point of being able to speak, walk, and regain their functionality. *Inside Coma* presents their stories, along with startling research and developments in the fields of psychology, medicine, and alternative healing methods, which help us to understand and relate to the experiences of those in coma. Here we teach you powerful interventions to help your patients and your loved ones awaken their consciousness while in the coma state. This book helps shift the field of coma treatment from working primarily with healing the body, to healing the whole person, mind, body, and spirit. This shift offers tangible hope to those in these states, to the professionals who work with them, and to their families and loved ones. It advocates for a new ethical sensitivity that gives our patients and loved ones a right to be treated like human beings who continue to have sentient experiences.

Both of the authors, Pierre Morin and Gary Reiss, have been active in this work for more than 15 years. Gary has spent hundreds of hours helping to develop and apply these techniques with coma patients all over the world, including in the United States, Israel, Switzerland, Cyprus, and England. Gary has taught families and professionals worldwide how to work with coma patients by using this method. He has worked extensively with developing a hands-on approach to this work, and he also brings in his experience as a family therapist and organizational consultant. Coma Work is a combination of working with the person, the family, and the medical system involved with the patient's care.

Pierre Morin has worked extensively in the field of brain injury rehabilitation. He was the assistant clinical director of Switzerland's lead rehabilitation clinic for head traumas. He had the opportunity to implement the concepts and skills presented in this book in the therapeutic program for brain-injured patients. He worked individually with people in comas and taught the medical staff and friends and relatives of the patients some of the sensitive communication skills that are presented here. He currently assists individuals and families that live through a coma experience, and he coaches care teams on how to best support the individual recovery process.

Throughout this book, Gary and Pierre will alternate speaking about their personal experiences and their theoretical thoughts.

Pierre: Erin had been hospitalized for quite a while in the neurology rehabilitation station where I was working as an assistant clinical director in Switzerland. In a suicide attempt she had shot herself in the head and severely injured her brain. Her family told us that before her injury, she had lived in an abusive relationship and had experienced severe depression. Her brain injury was extensive—to the point that after several months of being unresponsive, she was diagnosed as being in a persistent vegetative state, a medical diagnosis that characterizes people as having no subjective experience or awareness. Erin showed no reactions to her environment, had no spontaneous movements, and did not respond to any of our attempts to stimulate or communicate with her. Most of the time she lay motionless in bed or sat in her wheelchair with her head hanging down. Her situation was dismal and very challenging for the whole rehabilitation team and her family.

I had just started my training in Process-oriented Coma Work[3] and with a colleague had started to work with my patients using my newly acquired skills. For more than six months I had had minimal success with any of my attempts to establish even some communication with Erin. Despite the lack of progress I continued to attune myself to Erin's world and to follow her minimal cues. In one of my meetings with her I noticed Erin's head posture and decided to support her head with my hands. In a gentle voice, I encouraged Erin to trust and follow her inner experiences. Erin showed no outer changes and reactions, and after 20 minutes I decided to turn my attention to another patient. I told Erin I would slowly take my hands away and take her back into her room. As I actually withdrew my hands from supporting Erin's head, she lifted her head and looked directly at me with a big smile. This brief and intense connection was to change my whole belief system and thinking about coma and vegetative states.

Unfortunately Erin's reaction was not repeated and she withdrew again into her remote and unreachable state. Nevertheless this experience was so strong that it forced me to reconsider my understanding of her condition. Erin's reaction was not compatible with my medical thinking and judgment that denied her any consciousness or inner experience. It launched me into a journey of researching and discovering new ways of conceptualizing coma and remote states of consciousness and advocating for a more differentiated view of, and therapeutic approach to, these enigmatic processes. Whenever I share this story with an audience it touches many of the listeners. Erin's story is my motivation for writing this book and I hope it will help us co-create a new collective attitude toward coma and remote states of consciousness and toward the people who experience them. I hope it will help advocate for a new ethical sensitivity that gives our patients and loved ones a right to exist beyond the mere vegetative condition.

For decades, doctors have assumed that patients who have been diagnosed as vegetative were like zombies and had no meaningful experiences or capacity for conscious thought. But recently, with the help of new functional brain scanning technologies, researchers have discovered that comatose patients are able to recognize the faces of family members, understand the dual meanings of ambiguous sentences, and perform complex tasks such as imagining playing tennis. These are patients who are, like Erin, lying in bed without any observable reactions to their surroundings, and up until now they were thought to have lost what makes a human life meaningful. In recent years, however, we have realized that people in these states are able to hear and understand instructions, retrieve a memory of a sport activity, including the concepts of what is involved in that activity, and keep their mind focused on that activity long enough for it to light up in a brain scan. In other words, they are still having meaningful experiences and are able to relate to the external world as well as their own inner world.

The experience I had many years ago with Erin changed my world view and launched me into a quest to research new treatment approaches for patients in coma. My beliefs and struggles against the hopelessness in coma care are now being confirmed by recent scientific discoveries.

Concepts of illness and health are constantly shifting through the incorporation of older ideas from rediscovered ancient health traditions and newer ideas introduced by medical and scientific discoveries about the body. For example, in the 1940s germ theory strongly influenced notions of hygiene toward protecting oneself from external invaders. Later, increasing knowledge about the role of the immune system shifted the focus from the outside to what was happening on the inside. This has clearly influenced current interest in nutrition, vitamins, and trace minerals as immune modulating factors and agents.[4]

The late 20th century is best regarded as the molecular age of clinical medicine. The ongoing scientific advances provide detailed and precise knowledge of the workings of the human body at the molecular level. Most recently, much progress has been made in the field of neuroscience in regard to the structural aspects of the brain and its function. The developments in neurocognitive imaging (functional Magnetic Resonance Imaging [fMRI], Positron Emission Tomography [PET] scans, and the like) have made some of the workings of the brain accessible to observation. With increasingly detailed knowledge of the brain's activities, it looks like science will help us understand the biological pathways through which emotional, environmental, and social factors have their effects on the body. For centuries scientists and philosophers alike have wondered how mental thoughts cause physical actions or how exactly brain processes produce conscious thoughts and how those thoughts are performed in brain cells. One lasting question is whether the mind runs the brain or if the brain runs the mind. Even if many of the boundaries between the body and the mind remain elusive, increasing understanding of the brain's functions will help us to understand how the mind and body connect.

Estimates suggest that there are approximately 35,000 Americans in a vegetative state and another 280,000 in a minimally conscious state—a less severe condition, in which patients show inconsistent evidence of deliberate behavior. The total annual cost for the care of these patients in the United States is estimated between $1 billion and $7 billion. There are various different causes of these so-called Persistent Vegetative States (PVS), such as traumatic brain injuries or non-traumatic injuries from a stroke or lack of oxygen after a heart attack; degenerative and metabolic brain disorders, for example in Alzheimer's and in the process of dying, and severe congenital abnormalities of the central nervous system.[5] Most of these patients barely survive in nursing homes without any rehabilitation therapy. Insurers who base their assessments on the probable chances for recovery often assume that there is no hope for any improvement and will not pay for therapy. Families have no other choice than to place their loved ones in nursing homes where they will inevitably fulfill their role of "vegetating."

Currently, much about coma and the paths toward recovery—and the neurological developments that are driving it—remains a mystery. Many of the new discoveries allow us to separate the different states and levels of consciousness and to deepen our understanding of the brain's functioning; my skeptical mind motivates me both to follow the latest scientific developments and conduct my own research. The connection between the anatomical brain and the subjective experiences of our minds remains elusive. Many of us would expect that a severe brain injury would also destroy the ability to process information and relate to the world. Without my many experiences with patients like Erin, I, too, would have remained a materialist, but they have forced me to reconsider my philosophical assumptions about the body and the mind and to take a more sentient view. We do not yet have the detailed knowledge that would help us understand and interpret the extraordinary powers and qualities of the mind, many of which I now think remain alive in these remote states of consciousness. Many researchers are engaged in scientific endeavors to fill the knowledge gaps. In the meantime, it is our ethical responsibility to provide the best care possible to our patients and loved ones.

In my own experience, there is much more to discover about what we need to do to support the healing powers of people who are currently trapped in unresponsive bodies. This book attempts to fill this gap and introduces body-oriented treatment and communication tools for people in comas. Our approach is based on the inspiring work of our friends and teachers, Arnold and Amy Mindell, who introduced us to the idea of using both our awareness and a natural understanding of life as a process in constant change, as a way to work with people in various states of consciousness. This method, which is called Coma Work, has been incredibly helpful in my clinical work. I have applied it with patients in coma as well as with patients who had reduced or altered cognitive abilities. I also use it in my work with people who suffer from various long-term health issues such as chronic pain. In addition it helps me to relate to my own deeply internal states in which I contemplate the stillness of an alpine lake or the turbulent motions of a stormy ocean on the Oregon coast.

Gary: Modern medicine focuses on taking care of the body of the coma patient, as if the body is the only part left to take care of. Yet, the latest developments in medical research, and in Process-oriented Psychology,[6] show that people in comas are much more present than just their physical bodies. In this book, we present modern scientific research, Process Work theory, and stories from our clinical practice that illustrate our ability to connect with the whole person—mind, body, and spirit.

For many years, coma care has made a clear split between the person in coma and the person in waking consciousness, and not much has been done to address the whole spectrum of awareness. Those of us both in and out of coma are all at different stages on the awareness, consciousness spectrum. The techniques of Process-oriented Psychology can be used with anyone in any state of consciousness to help them become more aware.

This book builds on the pioneering books *Coma, Key to Awakening* by Dr. Arnold Mindell,[7] and *Coma, a Healing Journey* by Dr. Amy Mindell.[8] In his foreword to *Coma, a Healing Journey*, Dr. Arnold Mindell[9] describes where coma therapy is currently. "If we remember that, in the words of medical experts, today's medical treatment for coma is still in the dark ages and bound to improve in the near future, the kind of explicit, detailed, and compassionate communication Amy's book leads us through will stand independent of time."[10] I am convinced that modern science, and mind, body, and spirit-based psychological techniques like those from Process-oriented Psychology, together with the ancient, ongoing wisdom of indigenous shamanic healing methods will help take working with coma to a whole new level of success in reaching people in comas, and helping guide them through their journeys in coma land.

Why learn about coma? Well of course, if you are a professional working in this area, it is always helpful to learn new methods that may benefit your patients. But what if you are not a professional? Why read a book on coma? First, many of us will either have a loved one, or may ourselves be in coma sometime in the future, and knowing how to work with these states can be literally life saving, and it can also help us guide people into dying more consciously and peacefully. Secondly, learning Coma Work teaches us inspiring ways to work with our own waking consciousness and a way to be sensitive to others. In this book, we cover both aspects: how to work with others, and how to use coma awareness to change your waking life. This is similar to what the Tibetan Buddhists explore in *The Tibetan Book of the Dead.*[11] It is both a guide for how to work with the dying, and a guide for how to live a more conscious life. Learning to work with people in comas teaches us body and nonverbal signal awareness that can also be a source of wisdom for our own well being. If you learn how to follow subtle nonverbal signals, this may not only help you with a loved one in coma, but may also help you to be a more sensitive communicator and even a better lover.

How many of us will be touched directly by coma? Amy Mindell says in her book *Coma, a Healing Journey,* that at any one time, just in the United States, "there are 4,000 to 10,000 children and 10,000 to 25,000 adults in long-term coma (or persistent vegetative states)."[12] She goes on to say that there are approximately 500,000 new cases of head injury (one of the leading causes of coma) per year in the United States, and that 25 percent of these are categorized as leading to a persistent vegetative state. If we include all those who go into coma as part of the dying process, the numbers soar. Then we also have to look at all of those whose loved ones are in coma to have an overall picture of how many people are directly involved in and touched by coma at any one time, and all this is just in one country. So some day you or one of your loved ones may be in these states. The information in this book may save you or your loved one a great deal of suffering by giving you more information and methods for working with them. Coma and head injury can mean terrible suffering for individuals and families. It can mean months or even years of being in hospitals or various kinds of care situations, and loved ones may also have to take on a new full-time focus for their already busy lives. Coma can mean financial ruin for families, as the expenses of such extensive medical care can be tremendous. I have known families who were over $1 million out-of-pocket a year to give the best possible care to their loved one. Yet out of all this suffering, there is tremendous hope that out of the coma will come transformation and awakening: of self, loved ones, and everyone the person in coma touches.

One of the first questions families ask me when they contact me about Coma Work is: What can I do for their loved ones? They ask me if I have ever worked with someone in a similar situation who came out of coma. At this point in my career, most of the time I say yes. I tell them that of those I have worked with whom are given little or no chance of recovery, at least 35 percent have come out of coma. And, I also have to be honest and say that my goal is to help bring awareness to the person in coma. Awareness is different from healing. Awareness means that what happens is out of my hands. I am there as a facilitator of process so that the coma person can have the best chance of being in tune with what is happening and can gain something from the experience. This may lead to many different outcomes—partial awakening, staying in the coma, full awakening, or getting worse or possibly dying. Yet, at times, moving toward death can also mean freedom from being trapped in coma forever. People who believe in God will often say something like, "I understand that it isn't up to you, but up to God." Whether we call it following awareness or following God, it is clear that Coma Work is in a different realm from more mainstream medical or psychological methods. It is in the realm of the unpredictable, beyond the normal indicators of what is possible for recovery. If you or your loved ones are willing to journey into the realm of awareness, great learning and growth can occur.

It may appear that emphasizing awareness rather than healing makes these into two different directions, but my experience is that using this awareness-based method has given us the best track record I know of in terms of recovery. My work with clients over the years has shown me that openness to experience, and the learning and growth that seem to come from it, have a strong correlation with healing. When I applied an awareness-healing approach, many of the clients I worked with chose to go into the unknown and to find out, with awareness, what is possible. I always start by asking what the medical prognosis is. This is important information, but it is only the beginning of a broader picture. It tells us what is probable without mind-body interventions, but not what is possible.

In his appraisal of where mainstream medicine is currently, one of the top coma doctors in the world said that the hospital he was head of took fantastic care of the physical body of the person in coma, and that was it. The rest was up to nature. I appreciate all of the wonderful physical interventions that modern medicine can make. Without these interventions, many of the people I work with would not be alive and so would not have the opportunity to work with their comatose state. However, when I walk through the head injury wards, I see people left alone, and if their eyes are open, they are often just staring at the ceiling. Their only interaction may be when the nurses change their diapers or give them some kind of medicine or food. Often medical professionals will present families with statistics about their loved one's chances of survival and recovery and ask them to make huge decisions about termination of care without much professional interaction or support. Yet, I have had repeated experiences with patients who were given 0 percent to 5 percent chance of recovery who have gone on to recover their ability to speak, walk, and even return to school or work. How do we explain such apparent miraculous moments? One of the challenges for those of us doing mind-body interventions with patients is to create research that shows that the results are very different from those patients who were just given good medical attention. Nature can be assisted in healing, and as coma workers we are facilitating the natural healing of the person in coma. As a coma worker, I am also part of nature, so that just leaving someone alone to let nature takes its course denies them the crucial help they may need to turn the corner in their path to awakening.

Dr. Arnold Mindell in *Coma, Key to Awakening*, says that people in comas

are not simply brain-damaged vegetables in need of oxygen, suffering from the limbic lobe syndrome triggered by endorphins or like substances. Nor are they merely machines whose central nervous systems, stimulated by extreme physical states, produce haphazard hallucinations and visions. Rather, they are wakeful human beings going through one more meaningful step in their process of individuation.

In fact, people in comas resemble mythical heroes. Storytellers the world over have always enchanted us with tales of the shaman, the king, and the hero, figures who journey through the outermost gates of reality seeking information in the unknown reaches of existence to return with a divine message for the rest of us.[13]

In this book, we will tell the stories of these heroes who journey into the unknown to find their wholeness for themselves and for the rest of us. We will also talk about the latest scientific breakthroughs that help us understand this journey, and about how what we do as Process-oriented coma workers helps with this sacred journey.

Chapter 1

Recovery and the Process-Oriented Approach

In this chapter, we outline the foundations and underlying principles of Process-oriented Psychology that is the basis of our approach to Coma Work. We explain the initial steps for using this approach, and describe how it relates to working with coma patients and their families.

Process-oriented Coma Work is a method that was developed by Arnold and Amy Mindell (PhDs). The method helps establish communication with patients by picking up their subtle body signals, making them stronger and then following them. Process-oriented Coma Work differs from other methods in that it assumes people are not "lost" in a vegetative state, but can be reached by sensitively tuning in to their worlds, resulting in a method that is both deeply ethical and humane. The method can be learned and applied by family, friends, and professional caregivers.

We will interweave stories of some of our coma clients and their families and theories that explain our ideas and methods. Throughout this book, we will give our own personal perspectives. Pierre will share his experience from a medical viewpoint and Gary his knowledge of family and social dynamics. We include individual and partner exercises that are easy to follow and that teach the family and caregivers practical steps that they can immediately use to improve their communication and relationship to their loved ones.

Pierre:

It is important to emphasize that if we do not see responses in a patient, it does not necessarily mean that they are not aware.[1]

According to a 2001 study, between 40 and 60 percent of patients treated for head injuries in the United States are not properly treated[2]; moreover, since the mid-1980s, specialized rehabilitation beds for the brain injured are becoming scarcer. Many mildly to moderately brain injured people are denied treatment, and many who are severely injured and survive are left to vegetate in care facilities and nursing homes.

JULIE AND HER SISTER LESLIE

One day last September I received an e-mail from Julie.[3]

I got your name from Amy and Arny Mindell suggesting you might be able to help with my sister Leslie. My sister has been in a partial coma since June. I have read Arny's book *Coma, Key to Awakening*[4] and am very inspired. I can communicate with Leslie to a certain point. She can hear, move facial muscles, and she keeps eye contact when I am within a few inches of her face.

Julie continues to describe Leslie's condition and story and ends her e-mail with: "Is there anyone in our region who does Coma Work?. . . . I would appreciate any and all help. We want to bring her home but need to jump some hoops. I am not sure as of this last visit if she wants to stick around or not. . . . I would appreciate hearing from you. Julie."

This is a typical e-mail from a family member who is desperate to get help. Julie feels abandoned by a medical system that focuses on the body's needs and is helpless in addressing the emotional and spiritual needs of patients in comatose states and their families. Julie is encouraged by Arny's book and looks for additional help. This e-mail was the beginning of my journey in trying to help Leslie, Julie, and their whole family. As many similar families are who take care of a loved one in coma, they were desperate. Rehabilitation programs and specialty hospitals are inaccessible, and only a few states are capable of providing even the most minimal level of specialized care. To qualify for a rare post-acute brain rehabilitation bed, patients have to show that they can respond to commands like asking them to lift or turn their head, move a limb, etc. If the patient meets these criteria, it starts a marathon of bureaucratic paperwork, struggles with insurances, and phone calls with administrators to get on a waiting list for an already occupied specialty bed! If the severely brain injured patient does not fulfill the minimal criteria, he or she will be shuffled out of the hospital and bounced back and forth from nursing home to psychiatric ward, from emergency department to group home and the care of their families.

Medical professionals and the patients and their families live in different worlds with different paradigms and world views. Doctors see a broken machine body that is unable to function and respond. Family members experience their loved ones in a traumatic state that makes it difficult to get through to them. They see some movements, facial expressions, and possible signs of some sort of contact, but they have no clue what their loved ones are experiencing. Are they suffering, scared, or lonely? What can we do to make them feel better? Families are left alone to research the Web and social services for anything or anyone who can help them make sense of what is happening to their loved one and to find minimal support. Most severely brain injured people, like Leslie and her family, are not getting much help. They end up neglected and isolated, relationships break up, and families fall apart. A challenge like Leslie and her family's is an upheaval of enormous proportions. It may shatter their worlds, physically, socially, psychologically, economically, and spiritually. Leslie's family was privileged enough to be able to bring her home despite her being on a ventilator and needing two medical caretakers around the clock.

In late December Julie wrote me again. The family had been able to bring Leslie home. She was still on a ventilator and fed through a tube. She needed continuous medical care from a team of nurses, physical therapists, and doctors. Julie, Leslie's husband, their daughter, and another sister were coordinating her care. We agreed that I would join them for a weekend, take time to work with Leslie, and then instruct the care team in ways to communicate with Leslie. This is how I came to meet Leslie, her family, and some members of her care team.

Leslie's Story

But first here is Leslie's story: Leslie (age 55) was an aerobic and Pilates instructor and a personal trainer for many years. Previous to her coma she was a practicing Spiritual Intuitive, taught Reiki, and had studied nutrition extensively, intending to become a nutritional counselor. Julie told me Leslie had amassed a remarkable knowledge of health and alternative healing. She was stricken with a series of physical ailments beginning in 2001 that culminated in a mysterious autoimmune syndrome that slowly manifested in different ways. Her digestive process was the first system to fail, followed by peripheral neuropathy that over four years took away her ability to walk without assistance. More recently she developed malnutrition as a result of not being able to assimilate the food she was taking in. She became allergic to a number of foods and lost considerable muscle mass, eventually weighing only 95 pounds. Her skin had become quite thin and susceptible to bruising. At times she retained inordinate amounts of fluids. In April 2008, she was admitted into the hospital emergency unit with heart failure due to her autoimmune disease complications and ended up in intensive care.

She was diagnosed with a rare genetic condition in which proteins are not processed correctly and, over time, accumulate and essentially attack different systems in the body. The allopathic medical knowledge of this rare disease is limited, as is its treatment. If caught at an early stage, it can be managed and liver transplants have been a successful cure. But for Leslie the doctors at the hospital admitted there was nothing they could do except to offer Leslie comfort care. So Leslie and her family turned to a naturopathic doctor for assistance.

The naturopath started Leslie on a regime of natural supplements and enzymes to address her condition from the cellular level. The goal was to rebuild her stomach and digestive tract, while eliminating the proteins that had been ravaging her. Leslie made remarkable improvements and was able to wean herself off of the ventilator. She was then transferred out of intensive care to an interim hospital for further rehabilitation.

While she was at this hospital, a mistake was made. Leslie was still not able to swallow and was receiving food through a stomach tube. Leslie was given an excess of protein, which caused her heart to fail. She had to be resuscitated and suffered some brain injury due to lack of oxygen. Since this severe trauma Leslie has not regained consciousness and is in a partial coma.

Julie and her family had spent many hours reading to Leslie, massaging her, singing to her, and helping the nurses to turn her. The family insisted in taking Leslie home to a house they had recently purchased. It took quite a bit of convincing to get the hospital to agree to support the family in this goal. Caring for someone in a coma and whose breathing requires the support from a ventilator requires high technical skills. But Leslie's family was extremely motivated. They hired a care team, and in November 2008 they were able to bring her home.

At home Leslie made steady progress on a lot of levels. She gained weight and started to turn her head on her own and tracked people with her eyes. Her family believed she was able to see and hear. Leslie's care team consisted of an anthroposophic and allopathic doctor, a nursing staff, and caregivers. Her husband, Peter (age 58), was deeply committed to her care and was by her side most of the time. Julie visited every two weeks from five hours away and stayed three to four days as a backup. Peter's daughter, Dawn (age 34), lived right around the corner and was extraordinarily supportive.

This is the information I had when I first met with Leslie. I had been in contact with her sister for about five months. Leslie's story impressed me for her resilience in fighting what seemed to be an uphill battle. She had been an alternative health leader in her community and admirably able to overcome many of her challenges. I thought to myself that her health leadership might have been related to her at first unclear health issues. She possibly knew something was wrong and was trying to help herself ahead of time. Unfortunately the high protein nutrition she received in the hospital was poison for her and led to heart failure, resuscitation, and anoxic brain injury.[5]

When I first visited her, Leslie had been in her current state for about 10 months. She was in a bed in the middle of the family room. She was being breathed through a tracheotomy incision by a noisy ventilator and had several IV lines. She was half sitting up, with her eyes closed, and her hair was hanging over the pillow. Her mouth was drooping and her cheeks were relaxed. She was dressed not in a hospital gown but in a pretty shirt, sitting up, and obviously in an altered state. Her eyes were open but there was no clear sign that she was looking at something or making contact with her environment.

Our Meeting

What follows is a narrative of my first interaction with Leslie. I am shifting into the present tense to convey my experience of the actual work.

I am nervous going in to see Leslie, knowing she had had a heart attack and not knowing how strong her heart is. I know that she sometimes develops edemas in her legs over night, which indicates to me that her heart is still weak, so I know I need to be quite cautious and gentle in how I interact with her so as to not to excite her too much.

As I am approaching Leslie I notice her breathing and in the rhythm of her breathing I gently introduce myself to her as someone her sister has invited to work with her. I tell her I am there to assist her, to meet her where she is, and to follow her direction as where to go from there. Leslie's eyes open slightly, she shakes a little and I encourage her to go ahead and do what she needs to do. Her eyes move more and they try to make contact. I notice that her eyes are not synchronized and that one eye is focusing more than the other. She seems closer to the "surface" than I anticipated; she definitively hears and is possibly seeing, at least with one eye. Then she has some more little jitters, sighs, and her breathing changes (though she is on a ventilator, Leslie is also partially breathing on her own). Some of these somatic feedback reactions to my communication look like positive feedback to my approach. I hesitate, uncertain about my assumptions, needing to check them out, so I take a step back to see if something changes, but Leslie doesn't seem to relax when I am further away, so I move toward her again and her eyes open up again.

This eye opening suggests to me that Leslie has partial control over her eye movements. Negative feedback from her would be to close her eyes more instead of opening them more. If she were reacting negatively to me I would expect her to shut down more rather than showing more reactions. The notion of feedback is very important when you relate to someone who can't tell you directly that they don't like what you do. One way comatose or verbally unresponsive people communicate negative feedback is by pulling away and withdrawing. Many of us who *are* able to talk but have difficulties giving direct feedback will do the same. We may change topic, look away, or become silent, thus communicating passively that we don't like the direction of the conversation! Similarly, that's how comatose people communicate displeasure. In my experience they leave, they are less present, and they withdraw.

I decide to pick up on Leslie's positive feedback of opening her eyes when I move toward her, so I move closer and tell her I will touch her shoulder, the body part that was jittering. As I am touching her shoulder she seems almost to look at me. Then her body relaxes, her eyes close, and I encourage her to take a break and follow her inner experiences. I stay with her, pacing her breathing, and after a few minutes, while she opens her eyes again, I say: "Hello, this is me, Pierre, nice to meet you." She looks back at me and then her eyes turn upward with a fixed gaze. I wonder if she is having a partial seizure[6] or if she is seeing something intensely. Shortly her eyes come back down again and she relaxes back. I think to myself that she became excited and that now she might be tired again. Fifteen minutes have past and thinking of her heart and because of the excitement I step back to give her space to take a break. From the perspective of awareness and consciousness I would love to support her excitement more, but until her heart is stronger I am going to go slowly with my interactions. Leslie has been lying in bed for months and her body has become quite weak, and any little excitement requires a lot of energy.

Later I ask Julie to join me, and I observe her interaction with Leslie. Leslie responds to her as well and I can see that they have a close connection. Julie seems shy to get close, probably because I am there, so I encourage her to get closer. I explain to Julie that because of the communication barrier, a lot of people in Leslie's state develop a kind of *locked in syndrome*[7]; they pull away and become afraid of the world. I tell her Leslie looks like she needs a lot of close contact. Closeness, intimacy, and body contact are in general very important for comatose people. They are already very separated from the world around them and need us to breach the distance and reach out to them. In addition I know from Julie that Leslie is a physical woman and likes yoga, so I suggest to Julie that she practices yoga breathing with Leslie, touching her gently and following her feedback.

In a break Julie and I think together. We both agree that Leslie seems closer to the surface than she is able to vocalize, and that she might understand a lot. I suggest she may be locked in, in a psychological sense, hopeless about making contact. We wonder how tough it must be to make contact through something like a glass wall. Leslie might like to come out. But it is difficult for her. Like most of us, her family and friends are shy around body contact and don't know how to relate nonverbally. We all need encouragement to overcome our contact shyness around people who are in altered and unresponsive states.

As I work with Leslie and her caregivers, I observe how rapidly they move. They are well meaning and interact with Leslie at a normal tempo using rapid motions and interactions. The experience of time and motion changes in coma. The brain's ability to process sensory information is altered. Within the same way that getting closer is helpful, slowing down also seems to work better when you relate to someone in coma. With Leslie's family and caregivers I take time to watch the videos we have taken of our work with Leslie and then we discuss the reactions we see to various interventions and contact styles. Later we experiment with going slower, giving time for Leslie to feel and react. We practice centering ourselves, slowing down and tuning ourselves into Leslie's state. We talk about contact shyness and intimacy and what feels right for everyone. And we discuss the difficulties we have, as caregivers, to be deep in ourselves while we are interacting, engaging in nursing activities, and communicating. We practice with each other various interaction styles and learn to appreciate how it feels to be touched in a certain way or another. We discuss the reality of our own extremely busy lives and our own needs. We discuss what Leslie teaches us about time and love, and about our own feelings. We develop ideas about how we can integrate her teaching in taking time with each other, sharing sentient feelings between family and care team members, and reconnecting with our deepest selves.

After returning to Oregon I went over my experience with Leslie and her family and the caregivers. When I re-watched the videos, the family's contact shyness once more caught my attention. I also noticed Leslie's outfit. The way we dress ourselves and our loved ones provides information about how we think we ought to be. Family expectations and dynamics can be experienced in many ways. Some are more obvious and are conveyed through direct interactions. Some behaviors are more subtle and are expressed in indirect signals. A possible explanation of Leslie being neatly dressed is that the family wanted her to be better, wanted her to be her old self again. This could also explain some of their communication styles that were very verbal. Negating the disability and the change of state is understandable from a family perspective that wants to hold on to the image of the healthy and normal Leslie. On the other hand, this can contribute to communication blocks. In the past I have had many discussions with care teams on this very topic. There is a value in relating to differently-abled people just like everybody else. You want to show respect and avoid patronizing people by treating them like "babies." Then again, keeping a conventional and regular communication and relationship style marginalizes the coma and altered state. The trick is to do both. Remembering the old self *and* getting to know the new person.

In my review of the tapes and in my feedback to Julie, I explored the possibility of setting up a *binary communication*[8] system to help solve problems or get answers from Leslie to some of the questions the family had. I recommended to experiment with Leslie's eye opening as that movement may be under control and to also use Leslie's teeth. To Julie I suggested that she wash her hands and put her fingers between Leslie's teeth and ask Leslie to squeeze, bite down her teeth slightly if she agrees to something, and not to bite if she doesn't. I advised Julie to first set up a consistent yes, and then ask yes and no questions. Leslie's jaw looked as if it was just hanging, but as Julie and I interacted with Leslie, she moved her jaw intentionally and with control. Many comatose people have only very limited motor control over any body parts. Finding the one little movement that is still under control can be tedious, but then it can be the door to the comatose person's consciousness and their capacity to relate.

With only anecdotal information about Leslie it is hard to know what her overall process is. We only know what she has been like in recent times. A further exploration could include information about who Leslie was as a little girl. What do her baby pictures show, especially when she was three to five years old? Is she shy or boisterous in the pictures? This early quality may be something that is very important to bring out more in the present. At early ages people are still themselves;

they are still their unique self, the way one is meant to be before one gets "squashed" by socialization processes. One way to look at development and individuation is that it is about rediscovering that old core self. This can be used in relating to comatose people. With Leslie we could "talk" directly to the essence of that little girl in her. The idea would be to fantasize into that girl's process as if that was mythic for her and then check her feedback.

Additionally, in my conversations with Julie I advised her to gather the family together outside of Leslie's room and take time to share what everybody is feeling. In one letter Julie had stated that: "In our wordless world we are the best of our better selves." So I suggested that Julie tell Leslie: "I wasn't perfect with you in everyday life; but I want you to know I just have a lot of love for you." My final thinking about Leslie's process was about the "smooch" part of life. I perceived the family to be shy around feelings and was thinking that Leslie was possibly a teacher about closeness and intimacy for the whole system.

I have retold Leslie's story and my process around it in detail to help illustrate what Coma Work is and can be. In this situation it was mostly about meeting Leslie and helping her family and care team to communicate with her. We can say the Leslie is perhaps doing well; although she is not present in our everyday fashion she seems to be in a stable, comfortable state without much sign of distress. Her family is struggling with the immense load of her care and with not knowing what Leslie might want. In this instance Coma Work included individual work with Leslie, Julie, Peter, and other members of the family and care team; relationship work between Julie and Leslie, and other care team members and Leslie; and finally family and team work. Leslie is the identified patient, but the whole system is in need of help and support. Thanks to her family, Leslie is getting extremely good medical care and a lot of specialized services. She is at the center of a hub of activities that surround her care and receives more attention than most people in comparable conditions. Nevertheless her care team experiences, as most of us do, a considerable sense of helplessness about the softer skills of connecting with a person in coma, relating to their state of consciousness, and interacting with them. Our busy lives lure us into focusing on outer pursuits and behaviors and marginalizing our inner worlds and feelings.

INNER AND OUTER EXPERIENCES

Process-oriented Coma Work is uniquely suited to assisting people in comas and offers tools to establish some communication with a person in an altered state of consciousness or with only a few remaining fragments of consciousness. Process-oriented Coma Work provides the methodology that allows us to promote the cognitive abilities that are still present and support the healing process. Using a person's minimal cues and behavioral fragments, we are able to unfold and expand their range of meaningful behavior and ability to communicate.

Below I retell the story of Mr. Matthias Turtenwald, adapted from Arny and Amy Mindell's Web page. His wonderful story demonstrates his lived coma experience and the difference between his inner experience and the observed outer experience. Together with the report of his friend, Theresa Koon, I trust it will give hope to those worried about comatose states.

Matthias Turtenwald's Story

On January 14, 1996, Matthias was alone at home with his three children. In the afternoon they decided to go to a nearby tower to see the sunset. They drove up there and climbed the tower. The sunset was very beautiful. Going down again, the two older children Stefan (age 11) and Felix (age 9) went first and Matthias followed with his youngest son Franklin (age 5). At the second level from top Franklin told him that he was scared about going on. Just to soothe him Matthias lifted him into his arms. At this moment he slipped and they toppled over the banister.

They both fell 28 feet and Matthias hit his head on the concrete. Franklin fell on his body. Matthias was immediately unconscious and was brought to a university hospital. A neurosurgeon performed an operation and thought that there was no chance for him to survive, or that he would survive only in a vegetative state.

It took six months until Matthias came back to life. Matthias remembers that he strongly felt the love he received during his coma from his wife and especially from a nurse who cared a lot about him.

In May, Theresa, a friend of Matthias, came from the United States and he remembers that he recognized her. He remembers reacting strongly to her English and the way she breathed with him. He recounts that his way of experiencing and thinking in the coma was very different from his normal way of thinking. He remembers some feelings he had during the coma such as a special scene from the film *Sleepless in Seattle* that he associates with his chances of recovery. After his coma he started at the level of a small child. At first he only understood English and not German anymore. It took him a while to learn German again. He didn't know that he had three children and he didn't know anything about the reasons why he was in the hospital. Being in the hospital felt normal to him.

Then his friend Theresa sent him Arnold Mindell's *Working on Yourself Alone: Inner Dreambody Work.*[9] When he read this book he started very slowly to understand that something had happened with him. It took him another year to understand everything and to really start his life for the second time.

Matthias's friend Theresa Koon's recounts her experience of her interaction with him. On January 14, 1996, Theresa had a dream about Matthias. In the dream, his feet were strapped to the wing of a plane, and he was flying that way, standing out on the wing. There was a sense that he might never land, that he might die, trying to fly like that. She first heard about Matthias's accident when she called the theatre sound studio where Matthias worked in Rudolfstadt the next day, wanting reassurance that her dream had no significance. Instead she was told about Matthias and Franklin falling from the tower, and that the doctors were skeptical about Matthias's chances of recovery. His wife confirmed this, although she remained hopeful throughout his long coma, the surgery, and a bout of pneumonia. When Matthias's condition was more stable, the wife asked Theresa to come and see what she could do to help him back to full consciousness. At this time the doctors still did not think that this was possible.

At the end of April, shortly before Matthias's birthday, she headed over to Germany. What she saw when she went into his room was not a familiar person. Matthias had been muscular, vibrant, and warm. The person she encountered looked limp, miserable, and lost. His head was crushed on one side, and although his eyes where open, no one was looking out of them. His mouth was slightly open, his lips curving sharply down in a frown. He would reach up with one fist and rub at the hurt part of his head, then roll over to one side, then back, then rub, then roll. There was no sense whatever that he recognized Theresa or even that he knew that anyone had entered the room. His wife spoke bravely to him, letting him know what a delightful surprise she had brought him. Theresa did not believe her arrival registered with him, at all.

She went over to him and brought her face down close to his ear on the uninjured side, and put her hand on his arm. She told him who she was and that her hand was squeezing his arm. She inhaled when he did and spoke while they exhaled, telling him what she noticed, or mimicking the sound of his breath. There was a dissolving of boundaries, like being an infant. It was a state that was easier and far more familiar than she'd expected, but it was also disorienting. She doesn't know how long that first session was, and doesn't remember what signs there might have been that gave her a sense of hope. She thought it wasn't anything tangible, at first, but she had the vague feeling that she'd connected with him in there and that on some level he knew someone was with him.

The next day she worked some more, and it seemed to her that his movements had some slight variation to them. When she spoke at his ear, she thought he "took it in" more. His breathing would change, and when she registered the change, he would change it more, so they had a little breathing dialogue, punctuated by supportive feedback from her. Matthias spent much of his time rolling back and forth; since he couldn't talk and they had no clear form of communication, Theresa recounts that she might have tried too hard to find meaning in his action. She thought she saw a struggle going on in him, some effort to work something out.

She told him she imagined that everything must seem pretty strange to him, and that she would try to keep him company where he was. Since she didn't know what he wanted for sure, she told him that whatever he wanted was all right, that she wouldn't try to make him do anything. Some things she said seemed to make him agitated, though she cautions that may only have been her desperate attempt at interpretation. However, his eyes were changing, and it was much easier to get his attention than it was on the first day. He seemed to look directly at her, as if he saw and heard her. Soon it was clear that he understood what was said. The aides who had been working with him were amazed at the changes, and they stopped in frequently to watch his latest accomplishments. One afternoon they had him propped-up in a wheel chair with a tray. While talking to Theresa, someone absently rolled a small ball across the tray and Matthias stopped the ball with his hand! He had seen it, registered its speed, and caught it. They all gasped, and had him do it again, then again. Then they gave him a magazine and a pen. He took the pen and wrote what looked like words, though they couldn't read them at first. He was clearly reacting to things that were happening around him, apparently for the first time in over four months.

One day Theresa was trying to play a tape on the cassette player, and though she pushed the "play" button, no sound came out. She explained her difficulty to Matthias, and he reached over and nudged the volume knob, which made her laugh, since his diagnosis of the problem was correct. On another occasion his brother brought him a present, and he helped open it himself, and turned the pages of the beautiful book, looking at the pictures. This was all done by a person who only days before had not really appeared to be conscious.

Theresa remembers what appeared to her to be the biggest turning point. The rehabilitation aides had put braces on Matthias's legs and, with the two of them to support his shoulders and two more to move his feet, they started to remind his body how to walk. He didn't have any muscle strength, but they were working with his brain by moving his legs. She was stationed at his ear, staying connected. It was so clear to all of them the moment his will joined with his body and he took up the task of walking. He was actually kicking his legs forward for each step, supported by the aides but definitely leading the way himself. As the six of them moved out into the hallway, a cheer went up from all the staff at the sight of this supposedly helpless case, more-or-less walking down the hall. At that moment his mother showed up with Matthias's brother Gunter. While they were there he swallowed food for the first time. It was a joyful day. Several months later, his wife Anett called Theresa in Oregon with the phone number for the rehabilitation hospital and asked her to phone them. When she did, she heard Matthias's voice on the other end, talking to her from his bed in English! He knew who she was and talked nonstop in a stream-of-consciousness way that was both magical and surprising. He had lost most of his memory. At first, he didn't know about the accident, his job, his family, or his own childhood. In conversation, it was difficult for him to stay on any one topic or remember what was said. The fact that his English came back practically intact was astonishing.

Over the next two years, much of his memory returned, and he was able to somewhat describe his coma to Theresa. In it, he said he had been at a point where he could have lived or died, that he had made the choice. Death looked like an appealing choice, but he wanted to live to take care of his children. He tried to choose life, but he couldn't find the way back to it. He couldn't take charge of his body. Then something happened to help him find his way. Though he mentioned her contribution she thinks his will was strong enough for it to have happened anyway, and Anett never lost faith.

In my experience, the extraordinary story of Matthias, Anett, and Theresa illustrates many aspects of the perplexing ways that a person can recover from what at first seemed to be a situation with a poor prognosis. It also demonstrates the limitations of current medical knowledge.[10] The brain remains a mystery. Why did Matthias wake up speaking English and not German? Medical literature describes a rare condition called foreign accent syndrome after strokes and brain injuries. In these patients, the brain injury affects the speech melody and rhythm, which in turn makes them sound as if they were speaking with a different accent. But Matthias had completely lost his understanding of German. Did Theresa's special communication skills have any influence on Matthias's understanding English and on his overall recovery? We will never know for sure in a scientific way. Nevertheless their experience and story motivates me to continue my pragmatic research about different ways to communicate with people in comas.

In the following paragraphs I will now develop some theoretical ideas and describe the various verbal and nonverbal communication skills that we use in Coma Work.

BODY LANGUAGE

Coma Work uses both conventional verbal communication as well as nonverbal communication such as body language. Body language, nonverbal behavior or nonverbal communication is usually understood as the process of communication through sending and receiving wordless messages. Nonverbal communication can occur through any sensory channel—sight, sound, smell, touch, or taste. It includes gesture, posture, body movement, use of time, and reactions to the use of space. Body language, or the minimal cues and micro expressions we give through body signals, often reveal feelings and emotions. They can be used to decipher hidden emotions and are extremely useful in relating to people who don't respond verbally.

Milton Erickson, a famous psychologist, acquired polio when he was 17. Unable to move and unable to speak, he developed a strong sense of the significance of nonverbal communication—body language, tone of voice, and the way that these nonverbal expressions often directly contradicted the verbal ones.

I had polio, and I was totally paralyzed, and the inflammation was so great that I had a sensory paralysis too. I could move my eyes and my hearing was undisturbed. I got very lonesome lying in bed, unable to move anything except my eyeballs. I was quarantined on the farm with seven sisters, one brother, two parents, and a practical nurse. And how could I entertain myself? I started watching people and my environment. I soon learned that my sisters could say "no" when they meant "yes." And they could say "yes" and mean "no" at the same time. They could offer another sister an apple and hold it back. And I began studying nonverbal language and body language.[11]

In his writing, Milton Erickson originally used the notion of subliminal hearing in connection with body language. He described it as the ability to observe, through sensory acuity, the minimal cues expressed in a person's behavior as a result of what the person is thinking. He thought the reading of minimal cues required close observation and that minimal cues should be first noted without interpretation. The minimal cue may mean one thing about one person, yet something completely different with another.

Lie to Me is a popular new TV series shown on the Fox channel that bases its stories on a team of criminal investigators' ability to read and interpret people's minimal cues to solve their criminal cases by discovering the hidden lies and deceptions. The team specializes in understanding body-language and minimal cues. In their mind, body language is transcultural. They think that body language expresses the same feelings in everybody and thus is open to interpretation.

In our work with unresponsive coma patients we adhere to Erickson's views of open-mindedness about body language. In coma or after a brain injury the body's motor functions can be severely impaired or altered. Some body parts can be paralyzed or affected by spasticity. When someone has only very limited ways to express themselves, he or she may use the parts that remain accessible to communicate with for much more than would be conventionally expected. Imagine being locked in a body that responds only partially and in very limited ways. Any movement of any body part can be used to reach out. Some of the movements may be more or less under control but it is often hard to know with accuracy which ones are.

Here is what one brain injury survivor said about how she felt. She describes how she relied on outside support and how important it was for her family to interact with her:

As far as being aware, I remember much of what was going on around me during the coma. My surroundings seemed like dreams based on the reality taking place at my bedside. It was very important that friends and family continued to speak and elicit responses from me. I needed their interaction, even their foresight to play music or turn on the television. I look back and believe that I relied on their hope and trust in prayer.[12]

This is another argument for attempting various communication modes with people in comas. Using both verbal and body language enhances the range of communication and the chances of connecting with a person who is injured and is in a sensitive place.

COMA WORK: HARD AND SOFT SKILLS

Intrapersonal and interpersonal skills can be split into two categories: hard and soft skills. Hard skills are more technical in nature, whereas soft skills describe more feeling-oriented skills. In Coma Work, hard skills include medical knowledge, connecting with the person in coma by pacing his or her breath, signal awareness, the processing and unfolding of minimal cues and other body language, and deep body work techniques. Additional Process-oriented hard skills include knowledge of relationship work and facilitation, especially knowing and understanding the roles that are in the field of a coma patient, his family and care team, and their beliefs and attitudes.

Soft skills are about emotional intelligence. They describe your ability to feel into the world of experience of the patients and their families and the way you relate to the patients' minimal signals in a feeling sense. Can you sense their feedback and anticipate when they need to rest and take a break? Can you see beyond their everyday identities and sense what truly moves them? Can you hear their stories and see the mythical threads that their lives have tried to weave? Can you open yourself up to non-local events and synchronicities?

The initial contact with someone in coma is very significant. Your mood, atmosphere, attitude, and tempo are all communication signals. You are conveying your beliefs, values, and hopes through intentional and unintentional communication signals. What you say, how you introduce yourself, how sensitive you are to the person's signals communicates your intentions loudly and clearly. The nature of the initial contact depends on the situation and the level of responsiveness that the person in coma displays.

Personally, I always start by asking someone who knows the comatose person to come with me and introduce me. When I enter a room I check the atmosphere, the environment surrounding the bed, and the monitors. I check for reactions, sometimes it is a slight rise in heart beat visible on the monitor, or an eye opening, or a turning of the head. If I see a reaction I greet the person and comment on their reaction. I might say: "Hello there, I am Pierre, nice to meet you. I see you sensed me, thank you for acknowledging me." If I don't encounter any initial reactions I will slowly approach the bed, tune into the comatose person's breathing and, matching the cadence of his or her breathing, I introduce myself and tell her my intention: "Hi, ..., I am Pierre, ..., I am here to spend, ..., some time with you, ..., I will follow your lead, ..., as best as I can, ..., keep noticing, ..., your own experience, etc. . . ." I might then ask the person's permission to touch the wrist and will pace the breathing by gently squeezing the wrist when the patient inhales and relaxing when he or she exhales. While doing that I continue to speak in the same rhythm and start checking on minimal cues.

This work takes time when you start doing it to allow you to tune yourself into the comatose person's state. You need to pace yourself and synchronize your breathing. After a while it becomes a second language; it starts to feel more natural and you can use it in any little interactions. At this point soft and hard skills have merged together. You use your feeling experience and apply your knowledge and experience of nonverbal communication and body language skills. Theresa described beautifully how she stayed open-minded and responded to Matthias's body signals. This helped her connect with Matthias and helped Matthias in his journey out of his coma.

Process–oriented Coma Work uses minimal cues in an open-ended way, without initial interpretation. Expressions of distress may be about excitement rather than pain. I remember working with a young man who had suffered a bad motorcycle accident. Before his coma he was very athletic. In his coma, his body was very tense and full of *spasticity*, which was a problem for his care and many thought that tension could hurt him, too. We were tempted to give him a lot of calming medicine. When I worked with him and engaged with him and his tension, a very intense physical interaction unfolded. Matching his strength that was restrained in his spasticity, I helped him use that energy to pull himself up and make a lot of sounds. A part of my soft skill at this moment was to understand that this young and very physical man needed his strength to be matched and met. The uncertainty of interpretation is hard to carry for the care team and many health professionals will easily fall back into administering calming or relieving drugs that can then reinforce the comatose person's sense of isolation and feelings of being misunderstood.

In Table 1.1 I list some possible minimal cues and behavioral fragments and ideas about how you can interact with them while responding to a comatose person's communication signals. As a family member, partner, health professional, or caregiver, you can use some of these skills to add to your communication repertoire.

Table 1.1 shows hard skills to apply in Coma Work based on signal awareness. Other hard skills are listed in the following checklist of Table 1.2. This checklist is meant to stimulate your thinking as a family member or professional caregiver. If you are a coma worker in training they will guide you and remind you of important points to remember. The terms in italics are explained more in detail in the Appendix.

From our work with people with long-term health problems, we have come to understand illness as a deep and meaningful process beyond everyday reality. The wisdom embedded in body sensations and symptoms speaks to a different level of reality that complements and expands our everyday experience. Throughout the book you will find examples of people who in their coma went through deep mystical and spiritual experiences. A medical or spiritual crisis often requires us to re-evaluate our lives and search for meaning in a different way. Serious illness can be a chance to reconnect us with a spiritual or larger dreaming process. To

Table 1.1
Minimal Cues as Doorways to Communicating with People in Comas

Respiratory rate	Is it erratic or regular, labored or light, deep or shallow? Breathe with the person in the same rhythm and pace. Talk to him or her following the pace.
Eye movements	Twitches and flickers. If the eyes move to one side toward the ears, the patient might be listening. If they move upward he or she might be having a visual experience.* Use subtle touch near the eyes or ears to amplify the sensory perception of these cues.
Skin	Changes in color and moisture. Notice them, speak to them, say something like: "I see that; what a deep experience; believe in what you feel." Use all signals as doors into the unknown.
Body language	Posture, movements of limbs, and muscle tension. Use body-work techniques such as touching the body part that is moving, helping the movement to complete, impeding the movement to raise awareness about the moving body part; use touch, pressure, massage to unfold the inherent meanings.
Vocalizations	Coughs, sneezes, unidentifiable noises, unintelligible speech. Add your own sounds and tones and follow the patient's feedback. Use music and tunes, hum and sing, use vibrating sounds on bony protrusions such as the wrists, knee caps, etc.
Atmospheres	Moods, your own reactions and feelings. Take them seriously with openness and curiosity. They might give you significant leads into the patient's process.

*These observations are borrowed from Neuro Linguistic Programming (NLP). NLP is a model of interpersonal communication that addresses the relationship between patterns of behavior and the subjective experiences (especially patterns of thought) underlying them.

readjust to everyday life can then be difficult unless we stay connected with these deeper dimensions of life.

Based on this experience we have developed methods of working with the patient and encouraging them to actively participate in his or her own healing process. By exploring and joining the deeper meanings of the altered or withdrawn states, we are able to affiliate with the client's own interest in healing and growth and gain his or her compliance. All the hard and soft skills I described above have this goal in mind. Using these skills we bridge the communication gap and have a better chance in enlisting the comatose person in his or her own healing process.

Table 1.2
A Checklist of Hard Skills

Referral	Who made the referral? Where did they hear about Process Work/Coma Work or you as a coma worker? Who asks you to work with whom? What is his or her relationship to the person in coma?
Intake	Who is in a coma? What happened? What is/are the medical reason(s) for the coma? How long? How deep? Where is the person now?
History	
Consensus Reality	What is the person's identity? Professional/family situation? Hobbies? Strengths/weaknesses? Stresses?
Dreaming	Other body symptoms, *altered states*, moods, drugs and alcohol issues, other altered states, relationship processes/conflicts, etc.
Essence	Favorite color, poetry, painting, music; favorite spot on earth, religious/spiritual beliefs, etc.
Beliefs and Values	What are the *roles and ghost roles* in the system?*
Present Status	Presence of paralysis, *contractures, spasticity,* activities, sleep cycle, movements, vision, other signals.
	Medical support: *tracheotomy, percutaneous endoscopic gastrostomy,* ventilation, medication (anti-seizure drugs), rehabilitation schedule (physical therapy, occupational therapy, speech therapy, etc.), complementary medical support.
Phone/E-mail Support	How are you available? How often? For how long?
Contract	What are you going to do (work with individual in coma, family/care team work, training)? Where? For how long? With whom? What is your fee? Does it include travel? Where will you stay? Who is in favor of you coming? Who might have some resistance/skepticism? *Authorization and Release.*
Coma Work	Meet with family/care team; building relationship, discuss hopes and expectations, changes since intake or last contact, medical concerns; discuss how you are going to work with the person in coma, who will be present, who will introduce you. Discuss videotaping. Take time to talk to everybody present, build relationships. Observe, be aware of posture, join, test limbs, mention experiential channels, comment on minimal cues, unfold and respond to signals, add sound, follow feedback, keep track of energy flow, take breaks, include others, speak to the room, notice

(Continued)

Table 1.2
A Checklist of Hard Skills *(Continued)*

	non-local events, track interactions in the room and relationship processes, track your own process, close up. Debrief after each encounter, get feedback, ask for questions.
Training	Train family/care team members to use Coma Work skills in their interactions. Watch what they do, how they interact; look for relationship *edges* in the way they interact. Help them to be more intimate, get closer. Discuss their observations and what meaning they assign to signals. Process family and care team dynamics. Help them practice on one another. Then go back to applying the newly learned skills. Supervise and debrief afterward. If it is possible, use videotaping. Discuss books, resources, further training opportunities.
Follow-Up	Discuss follow-up before leaving. Tell the person in coma how you will stay in contact, if and when you are going to return. Make an agreement to check in with family and care team over e-mail or phone.

*See Appendix for an explanation of roles and ghost roles and other words in italics.

SOME STRUCTURAL BACKGROUND

This section compares Freud's structural theory with Arnold Mindell's conceptual framework. If you are a family member or if you don't like too much theory, you might want to skip the next few paragraphs. If you are interested in psychology or are a health care professional, this theory will help you compare some structural concepts and place the Coma Work ideas in the historical tradition of other psychological approaches.

Freud, the founder of psychology, was interested in the functions of the mind or psyche. His structural differentiation of the psychological mind into id, ego, and superego was an attempt to explain the intra- and inter-personal psychological dynamics he observed in his patients. His structure allowed him to develop the treatment methods of psychoanalysis. According to Freud's structural theory, the ego, the "I," or the autobiographical self, is the acting and organized part of one's personality and it has a conscious and unconscious component. The ego mediates between the id, the superego, and the outside world. The conscious component, which he called *perceptual consciousness*, receives sensory information and is in direct contact with the outside world. It is concerned with perception, reasoning, the planning of action, and the experiencing of pleasure and pain. It is conflict-free, operates logically, and is guided in its action by what Freud called the *reality principle*, which means it understands the obstacles of reality and is able to defer instant gratification. The ego's unconscious component acts through repression and other defenses to inhibit the instinctual urges of the id that are governed by pleasure and sexual and aggressive instincts. The ego also responds to the pressures of the superego, the largely unconscious carrier of moral values.

Arnold Mindell's Process-oriented Structural Theory splits the acting part of one's personality into a *primary* and *secondary identity* and the world of our experiences into *Consensus Reality, Dreamland,* and *Essence.* Our primary identity is that part of our identity with which we identify on a daily basis. For example, I would say that I identify with being a recent immigrant, a doctor by training, now a counselor, a husband, a father of a teenage stepson, etc. . . . And in addition, this Sunday morning as I am editing this book I would say I am a writer who wants to share his ideas, I am focused and concentrated on finding the right words and so on. The secondary identity or identities are the aspects of our personality and experience that we are less aware of. We encounter them at the fringes of our awareness through our night dreams, body experiences, conflicts, altered states, etc. . . . Just before I woke up this morning, I dreamed of travelling in a commuter train between Rome and Milan. The train was crowded with busy executives and office workers in their business suits and I couldn't find a place to sit. This dream shows me aspects of myself that I don't identify with and have marginalized. Italy is a country that I love and that I just visited two months ago. I love Italian food, but Italy is not who I am. My associations to Italy are about a sense of good life, enjoying friends, and food; it is about romance, romantic and passionate music, and the lush hilltop landscapes of Tuscany. I am also not identified with being a business executive. Just now I am marginalizing both my Italian and business executive nature.

Our primary identity gets its orientation from consensus reality: this is who we consent to be, what we do, what we believe and strive for. Our secondary identity is a marginalized expression of a dreaming process that balances the one-sidedness of our consensus reality and/or primary pursuits and concerns. The reality principle of the primary identity is expanded with an unconscious drive for a broader personal development toward self-actualization and self-realization. Parts of the secondary identity are disturbances that irritate us and make us self-reflect. Relationship pressures, body symptoms, moods, and complexes make us more aware and draw our attention toward increased consciousness.

Secondary dreaming processes move us to expand our present self and are an indication of our direction in life and thus a reflection of our future self. If I use my dream, my current personal development quest is about integrating my Italian traveler and business executive.

There are reasons for me to marginalize these aspects of myself. They somehow don't fit into my primary worldview of being a counselor and advocate of the poor and disenfranchised of our society, such as people in comas, refugees, and people with mental disabilities. I side with the current bad press that bankers have and repress my leisurely Italian nature in favor of my Swiss work ethic. This internal dynamic is characterized by psychological barriers and edge figures that defend these barriers.

In Process Work theory *edge figures* take the place of the superego. The edge figures are inner representations of collective values and norms. They protect the primary identity from the unconscious and challenging aspects of our personal and collective secondary processes. Using concepts of field theory Arnold Mindell describes the forces and powers of groups and communities, collective moods and atmospheres, as well as collective values and norms. They co-create the field and forces in which we live and the inner representations that shape our personal experiences and processes. My personal edge to embody Italy and the business executive as part of my own process is influenced by collective processes and norms that I was socialized with as I grew up in Switzerland as well as current social dynamics in my environment. My own inner struggles and development are part of a larger group and/or world process.

How does that relate to our work with coma patients? Process Work or Process-oriented psychology is *teleological* and believes that life is purposeful and meaningful. In extreme situations such as coma and life-threatening illness some of our developmental processes become more radicalized. For people in comas, their primary identities become less meaningful. On the other hand, supporting their secondary identities and processes has shown to be helpful. I always ask myself who is the person now? What do I sense is coming from him or her?

Process Work theory replaces the Freudian id with the concept of a *process wisdom*,[13] an organizing power that seeks to know itself through the diversity of the various conscious and unconscious experiences and tendencies in life. Process wisdom embraces primary and secondary identities and guides us in our developmental process. It resembles Bohm's interpretation of quantum physics and the concept of a pilot wave, which guides the motion of the elementary particle. Our path in life is guided by an intelligent principle. In Coma Work, childhood memories, stories, and pictures allow us to grasp the true nature of our patients, the person they were before they got socialized and the person they want to become again.

Mindell and Process Work further pragmatically divide the ways we experience consciousness into three levels: Consensus reality, Dreamland or dreaming, and Essence or Sentience. *Consensus reality* describes how a particular culture sanctions what is considered real. The concept of reality is a cultural concept, not an absolute truth. Communities need to agree on certain values and norms to be able to function. Without that, consent life would become chaotic.

Consensus reality also describes how certain experiences are deemed to be outside of the realm of social norms and are thus marginalized by most people. Currently mainstream science has a strong influence on what is perceived and accepted as objectively real, so people will tend to question the validity of experiences that are subjective, intuitive, and have no causal or scientific explanation. Many scientists reject dualism, that is, the separation between spirit and matter. How can something metaphysical influence brain matter and what are the physical laws that the soul follows? For many scientists every perception or experience must be traced back to a specific brain function. In the context of coma, for example, some scientists believe that if your brain is severely damaged, you are not supposed to be able to experience anything. In Chapter 2, Gary and I develop a new scientific paradigm that includes nonconsensual aspects of scientific reality such as subjective experience in comatose states, intuition, spirituality, and non-local events.

The second experiential level which Mindell calls *Dreamland* or *Dreaming* consists of experiences that elude our willful intent or agency. Dreaming manifests through your individual process as well as in relationship interactions and worldly events. Our body symptoms, many of our relationship interactions, the weather, our moods, and many of our emotions are not under our conscious control. These experiences are dreamlike and alter our intentions and our sense of self—our primary identity. From a Process-oriented perspective, they are a source of developmental wisdom. Coma and unresponsive states share medical or consensual aspects as well as dreaming elements. They have both medical and causal explanations, and experiential aspects that are subjective and dreamlike. Both Matthias's and Leslie's stories include dreaming qualities. Matthias's *Sleepless in Seattle* dream and Leslie's family shyness around body contact are examples of dreaming experience. They are meaningful in an elusive way and need facilitation and awareness to reveal their developmental potential.

Process Work defines the third experience level as *Essence* or *Sentience*. In *Dreaming While Awake*, Mindell defines this level: "Here you notice deep experiences, normally disregarded feelings and sensations that have not yet expressed themselves in terms of meaningful images, sounds, and sensations. These disregarded or marginalized feelings are sentient, that is, preverbal feelings and sensations."[14] It is the source of spiritual and creative experiences. It is the ground for experiences of unity, meaning, and direction. It is the experience of a guiding force that gives meaning and purpose to our lives. It is the essence of our being that is guided by our unique process wisdom.

In his book *The Quantum Mind and Healing*, Dr. Arnold Mindell lays out the fundamental Process-oriented approach that we take with the body and that underpins our Coma Work. Mindell calls this work Rainbow Medicine, and he says: "Rainbow Medicine includes the real time and space of physical reality as well as dreamlike levels of the body's psychological reality. Rainbow Medicine includes components of classical medicine such as anatomy, diagnosis, medication, surgery, biophysics, etc., as well as alternative medical procedures involving subjective experience, dream patterns, and all levels of consciousness."[15]

Process-oriented Coma Work addresses all three levels of experience. It includes caring for the physical needs of the body and the psychological, emotional, and spiritual aspirations of coma patients, their families, and their caregivers. Table 1.3 summarizes the Process-oriented Structural Theory and the definitions of the three experiential levels. It gives examples of their application in Coma Work.

Many facets of the processes that people in comatose and persistent vegetative states go through happen outside of our consensus reality world (see Table 1.3). Their movements and vocalizations are incomprehensible from a consensual perspective; but they can become meaningful if we address them from a dreaming and or sentient level.

As patients slowly begin to recover they often stay for long periods in altered states of consciousness or confused, withdrawn states that are closer to a dreamlike realm; they may speak in metaphorical analogies without *meta-communicating*[16] about them. Joining them in their experiential world, following and interacting with their signals and nonconsensual expressions is the door to discovering the possible meaning behind their experience. There is a deeply ethical dimension to this kind of approach. If you continue to relate to a person in such a state only from a consensual level, you in some ways deny their experience, you marginalize the person and his or her experience, you contribute to the isolation. An approach based on a different set of signals (minimal cues) is more appropriate and allows us to join the person in his or her state or inner experience.

By empirically differentiating between three levels of experience, Process-oriented Coma Work provides the basis for an integrative treatment for patients in persistent vegetative states (see Table 1.3). We think

Table 1.3
Three Levels of Consciousness

Consensus Reality/ Primary Identity	Culturally sanctioned aspects of reality and the way we integrate them in our identity. They include who the comatose person was, what he or she did, and how he or she identified him- or herself. They also incorporate conventional medical views and treatments of the body, but also regular nursing practices, like making someone comfortable, rehabilitative and palliative care, issues that need to be taken care of in regard to someone dying or being placed in a hospice, living will, advanced directives, etc.
Dreamland/Dreaming Level/Secondary Identity	Is our term for the field of subjective experiences, including unintentional processes in our bodies, dreams and images that accompany us throughout our lives, emotions and reactions we have to people and the atmospheres we sense around them. They give us indications about our secondary processes. In Coma Work we inquire about our patients dreaming experiences previous to their brain injury, their moods, relationship conflicts, etc. In the comatose state they manifest through minimal cues, behavioral fragments, and unintelligible utterances.
Essence/Sentient Level/Process Wisdom	Is the realm of the non-dualistic experiences and the process wisdom. Observer and observed, patient and caretaker are one unit. As an observer it refers to a state in which you feel your way into the person's altered states. It reflects an experience in which you have the sense of joining the comatose person in his or her world, rather than feeling like an outsider.

that all levels are important and can either be addressed simultaneously or alternately. For example, if you need to take care of a rehabilitative need (for example, as a physical therapist, if you have to apply a redressing cast to prevent further contractures or if as caregiver you want to make your patient or loved one comfortable), you can carry out the medical or care intervention and simultaneously remain aware of the person's minimal cues and behavioral fragments, relate to them and use them as feedback. Sometimes I have found that after I have briefly interacted with a patient's spastic posture and limb movements on a dreaming level, their muscle tension decreases and a medical intervention like the one mentioned above becomes easier to perform. If we train our awareness to enter dreamlike states, follow subtle body feelings, and notice minimal cues while also appreciating the everyday medical world, we can understand the consensus reality dimensions of a symptom like coma and remain open to other nonconsensual realities, too. The energy in a tense muscle is both a limiting process that needs to be treated for rehabilitative reasons and the expression of an innate power that may need recognition, guidance, and direction.

BASIC CONCEPTS OF PROCESS-ORIENTED COMA WORK

Gary: Pierre wrote in detail about the different levels of reality that Process-oriented Psychology addresses. These three levels of consensus reality, dreamland, and essence, are markers on the pathway of where our consciousness is at any given moment. When I work with a coma patient, I use this like a compass that I take out on a regular basis to ask myself where I am, where is my focus, and where is my client and their family. In Process Work I locate where I am and where my client is in two major ways. Pierre describes the basic steps we use to connect to ourselves and to our clients. Once this connection is established, my next step is to first assess what channel of perception the client is using. The main channels of perception I am going to work with are visual or seeing; auditory or hearing; proprioceptive or feeling body sensations and emotions; kinesthetic or movement; and relationship, which can be experienced in many channels. For example, I feel feelings for you and look at you; the world channel, where I am focused on my connections beyond one other person; and the spiritual channel, where I am having spiritual experiences. A map of the mountain is very different than the real mountain. In reality, the channels are mixed together, or often coupled. For example, now I am feeling and seeing. Sometimes channels are synesthetic, especially as we get down into the essence level. This means, for example, that I smell the color of the rose or feel the sound. Yet, asking my client and myself where we are in terms of these channels is still my main locator. The second locator is the client's level. Imagine you go to a large shopping mall to locate a friend. The channel is like knowing which store your friend is at; that is consensus reality, dreaming, or essence levels. The levels are like knowing what floor your friend is on. Now you might randomly run into your friend at any one moment searching for them, or you could just wait in the car and hope they come out and find you. However, having the basic information is going to increase the chances that you will find each other and have a successful meeting. Process Work coma methods are like searching with a global positioning system (GPS) locator.

My own style of Coma Work usually begins with consensus reality. I do an in-depth interview with the family members, and I try to find out as much as I can about how the person entered into the coma, what the medical prognosis is, what medical concerns I might need to know about while working with the client. Here are some of the basic questions I use when I am gathering information on the person in coma and their family, and that I think are important for caregivers to ask in making their assessments. Family members should be able to think about these questions as a way to help the caregiver make their assessment. I start out with consensus reality thinking in my questions and then go deeper into the other realms. Many questions mix in these different levels. The assessment helps me to begin to put together a theory of how this person's life was emerging; that is, how does the coma experience fit into the flow of the rest of his or her life. For example, if the person was depressed for years and flirted with suicide, how is this coma as a result of an auto accident relevant to this flow of life's experiences? Here we are looking for the connecting thread that relates the comatose experience to the rest of the person's life. My questions are also influenced by my training and experiences as a family therapist; I see the client as part of a larger system of family, hospital, and society in general.

Here are my general guidelines, some of which are the same as Pierre's and some reflect our different backgrounds, training, and style.

1. *Notice the family members you are talking to.* Sense the atmosphere. How are they? What is their attitude toward the person? Are they depressed, hopeful, etc.? How nervous are they about you coming in? What kind of pressure do you feel on you? What is their economic scene like, and is this a major source of concern for the family? Ask also what they are dreaming about the client. Notice the relationship of the family to the hospital system. Do they have generally negative or positive attitudes and relationships with the hospital and caregivers? How do they hold up and deal with the often-negative prognoses they get from the doctors? Can they believe in their own experiences with their loved ones? Are they in denial about the chances of recovery of their loved one, or on the other extreme, do they so buy into the mainstream medical model presented that it undermines their general feeling of hope? Does the family have religious or spiritual belief systems, and, if so, how do these support or hinder them in facing the current crisis?

2. *Gather the details around who is who in the family in terms of their roles, their attitudes, their levels of involvement with the client.* I especially look

for that one person who might be ready to step in and really take over my role. That is, I am looking for someone I can train and supervise to work directly with their loved one.

3. *Gather the details around the medical condition.* Details should include the medical state when the person went into coma, any progress that has occurred since then, the outlook for recovery, and any medical concerns that are present about you working with the person, for example, blood pressure concerns. My first principle is always to do no harm, to carefully know and respect the physical limits of my client.

4. *Collect information on how the coma happened.* Remembering the whole experience has a dreamlike nature, so for example, if it was an accident, exactly how it occurred, or if it was a stroke, what went on right before the stroke the last 24 hours before the stroke. Begin to think about dreamlike elements present in the accident. For example, if a young man is hit head on in an auto accident and flies out of the car, there is the violent impact of the accident, but also the flying that reminds me of a bird. There is something hitting, someone hit, someone flying, then someone coming down to Earth. This is important for me to know and then to ask the family more about. Was the person "flighty," needing to come to Earth, or overly earthy, possibly needing to fly more, or both. Were they full of fantasy and flighty in this way? Were they suicidal and trying to leave the Earth? How about all that violence of impact; what was their relationship to aggression like? How did life normally impact them and did they meet or impact life, head-on or indirectly? These all are part of my building a theory of who this person is, what they are doing in coma, and what might help them move out of this state. I will test this theory as I work with the patient and watch for their feedback to my theory and interventions that come out of my theory.

5. *Ask the family for details of what they have experienced with the person.* Details should include the general trends they have noticed, in terms of coming closer to awareness, going further away, staying the same, progressing then stopping at a certain point, etc. For me, the trends are as important, or even more important, than the specifics of what this eye or these arms do or whatever is happening. Is the client moving more and more toward awakening or presence, or further away. Did the client reach a plateau and when, or start going backward, and at what moment did this happen?

6. *What has the family noticed about changes in specific channels of perception?* For example, what new movements, eye movement and seeing; hearing changes and sounds; presence in relating and relationship in general are noticed? Do the eyes move more or less? Are they more or less focused and tracking? Does the person seem to be listening more or less? Are there new sounds they are making? How about their movements? Are they

moving more or less in general? Are their movements more or less detailed and coordinated? How is their body responding to touch and feeling? Do they seem to have more or less connection with their body feelings? How about relationships? Are they more or less interested in relationships in general? Are they doing anything new in relationships? These are just a few of the questions that are important to ask to be able to see not only the general trends, but also specific trends in specific channels.

7. *Ask about any big dream or big early experiences they remember about the person in coma.* In therapy with a waking person, I will usually wait for the first dream to be shared, or I may ask about a dream and especially the childhood dream or earliest experience remembered. The childhood dream is considered a foundation dream that shows very fundamental and deep patterns that a person will work on for a large part of their lives. Since the client is in coma, I will have to rely on the family to try and give me this information about client's dreams and childhood dreams and experiences.

8. *Ask about any other near-death experiences or being knocked unconscious.* I ask this because often there are other similar experiences present. For example, the last few people I worked with in coma had some other kind of coma-like experience through drug overdoses or suicide attempts. This gives me crucial information about who this person is and what their attitude may be toward coming out of the coma and back to ordinary waking life.

9. *Inquire about recent events around the time of the coma.* Ask about frustrations or other difficulties in the following areas: family, relationships, work, religion or spirituality, addictions, money, and any areas of struggle being their whole self. Are there parts of life marginalized; for example, are they always working and never play, etc? Are they always rational, never feeling much, etc.? I need to know who I am working with. This person is not just having a medical condition, but something relevant and meaningful to who he or she is. I am looking at both long-term patterns and short-term incidents that may be related to who these people are and what they are doing in this coma, as well as what their chances are of coming out.

10. *How was the person emotionally before the coma?* Was there any history or hints of depression? Was the person open emotionally? What feelings were marginalized? Most times when I address the depression question something comes up. I always ask was there any significant depression in the last year, or any pattern of repeated depressions? Often this question can be a window into the psychology of the person I am working on.

11. *How has the person been in the coma-vegetative state, that is, how do they appear to you in terms of their current identity?* How is this state a balancing or compensation for the pre-coma state—maybe the person is very active in this state and was very passive before? Do they fight a lot while in this

state, or are they passive? Were they generally a fighter or passive? Is this state close to their normal identity or very different and more like what we call their secondary process? Were they always a hard worker, and do they look like they are working hard to come out of the coma or do they look more like they are on vacation?

12. *As the final step in the assessment, take all of this information and make a theory about what the person is doing in this state, and what some of the pathways back to consciousness might be.* It is important to make a note of this theory, and, in working with the client at some later point, to test this theory. There are many ways we will cover to do this, from simply saying your theory to the client and watching for their feedback, to designing ways to test this theory. For example, if my theory is that part of what the person is doing in the coma is reacting to a life where they couldn't achieve the career they wanted, and the subsequent depression around this, I might experiment with this. If the person always wanted to be an artist and instead had to sell insurance, I might ask them if they could be an artist, might they want to come out of this coma. Then I would notice what happened.

We are moving toward a more process-oriented kind of assessment that includes, but is not limited to, the medical assessment. These kinds of questions are meant to balance the more medically-based consensus reality material we will run into. The most common descriptions of the person in coma are given in medical terms that describe the physical reality of the patient, and indicate how they came to be in a coma, the type and severity of the coma, and the possible chances for recovery. This consensus reality level description is all crucial information, and without all of this care of the physical body, the coma patient would of-ten have no chance of survival. However, working with the person in the comatose state, and helping the person move through these states to possible recovery, also requires working with the other two worlds of dreams and essence. Because these levels are left out of most traditional medical settings, it may be that we are only addressing one level of treatment—to address the consensus reality concerns that focus on keeping the body alive, but neglecting the other levels which may actually be the keys to recovery.

All of the statistics on rates of recovery are based on patients receiv-ing only physical treatment, so what those rates show is how much patients recover when given only physical treatment. When we go beyond this into the realm of psychological treatment, mind-body inter-ventions, and sentient-essence work, which is more in line with spiritual or transpersonal healing, then we are in a different kind of recovery program, and eventually we need to collect data on how people recover when given both physical healing and these other methods together.

This Process Work-based emphasis on working on all the levels is important because it also provides a different framing to the starting place of working with coma, viewing it not only as an illness but also as a doorway to meaning and transformation. This is why it is so important to present the stories of these amazing individuals and their journeys. As we move toward being able to present hard data on the differences this kind of work makes, it is also important to be able to present the human element for many reasons. The human element means this is not just a body in coma with these symptoms and this prognosis, but this is also Shirley or Carl or Jim or Stacey, and each of these people carry a story within them that the coma is a chapter in. Firstly, we can find ourselves in these stories; whether or not we are in coma, we all face similar challenges. Secondly, so often I get calls asking if I have ever had anyone who had a stroke who was told they wouldn't recover and who has come out, or whether I have ever had anyone come out after six months. The coma stories we tell give hope to those families through knowing that others have traveled this path and found meanings in this. Bodies and minds have been healed, and families and relationships have been transformed through the power of the coma and the healing journey it has inspired.

MOVING INTO THE WORK

It is important in working with people in comas to be especially careful not to hurt them physically, consequently undoing the medical healing that is being done. It is hard enough to follow feedback when working with someone who can verbally tell you what does and doesn't feel good. It is even more difficult with someone in coma, so I follow a few basic principles. First of all, I ask if there is anything that should not be done medically for the safety of the person. Perhaps they have an open sore, or an injury that I need to be especially careful with, or I may need to take care that if I am encouraging their excitement, that their blood pressure does not go up past a certain point. My second basic principle is to be gentle. Gentle here means that I am going to be careful with how much pressure or resistance I give someone. Even if I know that the part of the body is medically safe to work with, I am always aware that this client can't give me verbal feedback, so I will have to listen extra carefully to the nonverbal signals to make sure I follow my highest principle of doing no harm to my patients. I do interventions that are quite strong, but I always test and carefully work to that place of strength. For example, I might end up pushing down hard on someone's arm who is resisting back, and comment on how strong that person is, and I would work my way up to that level of strength, making sure I am watching for indications that I may be going too far or hurting the person or pressing too hard, and then proceed to higher levels of interaction, strength, and resistance work. It is very important to me that in the more than 15 years I have worked with coma patients, I have never as far as I know hurt anyone at all, and yet I am still careful. Part of that care is also that I am not only being careful for the sake of the client, but also knowing that this part of building a trusting relationship with the family and medical team is having them watch me work in ways that are both powerful and safe. Of course we are being watched carefully as families often don't care if we are mainstream (i.e., whether our methods are known and regular and familiar), but want to make sure that we are safe.

To understand how we do Process-oriented Coma Work, it is important to know about the basic principles of Process Work with symptoms that we use in our Coma Work.

1. *Cultivate a child's open, Buddha-like mind.* Use this to develop a curiosity and fascination with physical bodies that can take in all of the medical information and yet still remain open to the surprising things that are happening right in front of our eyes, even though they may not match the standard medical view. Develop the kind of mind that is open to all kinds of information, standard medical, Process-oriented, and your own dreams and intuitions.

2. *In the symptom is the possible solution.* If we go deeply into it, the symptom itself can provide us with the key. Otherwise it is like a dream unexplored. Exploring the symptom gives us the clues we need to understand what our being is trying to express and what directions the symptom is moving us in.

3. *Body symptoms are not just personal.* We carry with us our collective current experiences, our personal and collective histories, and sometimes our family history. We can find the current war, the Holocaust, our family issues, all in our body symptoms and experiences.

4. *Our bodies know best how to heal themselves.* If we can very closely follow our experiences and what nature wants to happen, then the healing will begin.

5. *A symptom is like a fixed state.* Going into the dreaming within the symptom rekindles an energetic flow in the body and allows the state to become fluid again and begin to develop.

6. *Work with all the channels.* Find the channel that is most active, follow that channel, and then let the work add on and expand into other channels.

7. *The sentient level is pre-dream and pre-symptom.* By going into the sentient level, it may be possible for us to step out of time and space, and then we can manifest the energy behind the symptom in a new way, rather than perpetuating the current expression of the symptom.

8. *Process Work is not for or against any particular type of medicine.* We follow the person's own process, unfolding their dreams and inner guidance, which at any given moment may lead us to do nothing, at another moment to see a naturopath or Chinese medicine person, and the next moment to consult a surgeon. All voices are important to the process, and we follow the client's feedback to see what is the right medicine at any given moment. People's processes call for different kinds of interventions at different moments. A true dedication to Process Work means giving the patient what he or she calls for, and not just what I as a practitioner believe is good or right. Outer caregivers reflect inner dream processes. Part of my process may need to have an outer surgeon with a knife reflect the knifelike consciousness I am trying to develop, or to have a shaman on the outside reflect the inner shaman trying to come forward. One of the reasons clients don't always follow a particular practitioner's advice is that they must be at the right place in their development to do this. For example, it is easy to suggest to someone that they should stop smoking or lose weight, but behind this decision are all kinds of feeling issues that need to be addressed before the person will be able to actually do it. The most helpful kinds of work often are to help the client to go back and forth between parts of themselves that are involved in the symptom. For example, with a client in ordinary consciousness, I might help them to go back and forth, to dance with the sides of themselves that want to lose weight with the side that says losing weight is like "giving into my mother's pressure to look a certain way and I say no to that." If one part of the client calls for surgery and others are against this, the surgery and recovery may not go as well. I have consistently had experiences with clients who have surgery, where we process the issues and the surgery thoroughly, who recover at rates much quicker than normal from the surgery. It is my idea that processing the issues around the kinds of treatments will not only show us the right treatments to follow, but make these treatments more successful. I believe this with a coma patient as well. For example, one client responded well to Process Work and to shamanism from a local indigenous shaman. However, his new wife wanted him treated primarily by her prayer group, and sent the shamans and process workers away. Her husband stopped what had been steady improvement. His feedback showed what method was right for him at that moment in time.

I started this section by talking about the way I locate people by using channel awareness. Whenever I get lost with a client, I ask myself are they seeing, hearing, feeling, moving, or relating? Then as I am working with them I also ask myself about the world and spiritual channels and how they are present. At times I also ask my clients these basic questions of what are you seeing, feeling, hearing, moving, or relating, and I watch their feedback. Sometimes it is obvious as the client is moving so much, making sounds, or relating to me or a loved one. Other times it is hard to find what channel, and I will search until I get feedback in one of the channels. The best way to learn to follow the different channels while working with someone in coma is to learn how to follow your own channels. I have talked in detail about the importance of these channels, saying they are the basic map for how to locate the client, and that I constantly return to this map when I get lost. Earlier I referred to this as my GPS. However, there are skills needed to follow channels. In Exercise 1.1, we learn how to find the channels, and how to follow ourselves in the channels, especially when we become stuck at places or reach edges—those places where we feel we cannot or must not move forward in that channel. Once you can follow the channels, then we will move on in the following exercise (Exercise 1.2) that covers how to go in and out of sentient awareness.

One of the keys to this inner work is knowing about the different possibilities of when you change channels. When a process deepens, it adds on channels. For example, if I am seeing and as I really look at something, I start moving, this is a deepening and allows for secondary material to come forward. However, if I am at an edge and my stuck point that comes up at the limits of what I identify with, channels may

Exercise 1.1
Learning to Follow Channels and Pick Up Edges

1. Close your eyes and take a few deep breaths.
2. Ask yourself, what channel am I in? Am I feeling, seeing, hearing, or moving? Follow the channel that you are in, and find a way to amplify this experience so that you begin to feel more, see more, hear more, or move more.
3. Stay with the experience until there is a channel change. For example, if I am seeing, I will work visually until I start hearing, feeling, or moving.
4. Now, take the process into at least one more channel. Notice when you come to an edge, and stay at that edge and process this until you find a way to go over it.
5. Once you are over the edge, let yourself explore the new place in your being with as much awareness and freedom as possible.
6. When this comes to some kind of completion, ask yourself how you can bring what you learned back into your daily life.

begin to flip. There is a different quality to this flipping, as I am no longer going deeper but staying on the surface by rapidly switching channels as I come up to edgy parts of myself. The best remedy for flipping channels is to go back to the original channel and to hold myself there until something changes.

This is the kind of inner work any of us can drop into at any given moment. The more this is done, the faster and deeper the work goes. For example, if I close my eyes now and ask myself what channel I am in, I am feeling this tightness in my back, probably in consensus reality from lifting some heavy objects; my muscles are tight. If I amplify this, I tighten my back and my shoulders go up, my face gets tight, my fists clench, and I notice I am now feeling and moving. My fists begin to pound the air and suddenly I begin to make sounds. As these sounds deepen, I am not only moving and feeling but making sounds, and I suddenly add on another channel. I see this shaman beating his drum, and he is doing a dance, like a bear dance, a white polar bear dance. I stand up and let him do his dance through me. He is beating his drum and doing a healing dance. I begin to feel into him even more and he tells me he is doing a healing dance for me, Gary, that I have been through a lot of work and beauty and difficulty the last few months and his drumming is bringing me back into my body more. I notice that I get to an edge and I stop at this point, so I will take myself back to this bear shaman. I stand up and go into this very strong dance with lots of sound. I complete this dance, and I have an insight. Those weren't just tight muscles in my back that I kept trying to loosen up. There was meaning in that tightness, there was a shaman's dance in that back. I have been very much in my primary process lately, having so much to take care of in ordinary reality. The shaman became marginalized and went into my back, and now that he did his dance and healing I feel more present and my back feels looser.

This is the same work I do with the coma patient. Yes, this is a coma on the physical consensus reality level, but who knows what shaman dances, what kinds of flying and being under the ocean and all kinds of dreamlike experiences are trying to come through this coma person. They are not just a person in coma, but I believe all physical symptoms are attempts to bring us closer to these other levels of dreamland and essence that we marginalize as individuals and as societies.

GOING FURTHER INTO COMA WORK

Dr. Amy Mindell, in her book *Coma, a Healing Journey*, spends an entire book on how to do the basic Coma Work interventions. She covers how to work in all the different perceptual channels. Her book is a great reference for how to amplify the different channels while working on the coma person. For example, she gives all kinds of different ways to work with different movement processes in the legs. In this book, I want to give some basics and then emphasize more how to work at the levels of dreaming and essence. I will take you there through theory, cases that illustrate the principles, and exercises that allow the reader to experience this for themselves. The easiest way to learn this work is to practice with someone who pretends they are in a coma. Both roles are training, what it feels like to be in coma, and how to work with the person in that state. In the next section, I present some of the exercises I use when I am training people to do this work. Some I have created myself, others I have taken or adapted from the work of Drs. Arnold and Amy Mindell.

Here is the first exercise (Exercise 1.2) to practice. These are the basic steps I use in working with someone in coma. There are two main steps. The first is to hook up with the client, to make a deep and strong connection with where they are. The second is to help unfold their signals in the various channels of perception by using different amplification approaches, and by following their process, your process, and the interaction between the two of you. It is best to practice with someone who will pretend they are in coma.

Exercise 1.2
Basic Coma Work Training

1. Have one person lie down and imagine he or she is in a coma.
2. The coma worker sits down next to the client. First, try taking a few breaths in harmony with their breathing. Next, in pace with their breathing, say something while using the following mannerisms: Speak on the exhales. Get close to their ear. Say something like this: "Hi. My name is Gary. I am here to work with you today in this special state you are experiencing. I am here to follow you; know that nature will best show us how to proceed. Believe in your experiences. Follow what happens and believe in what is happening. In a minute or so, I am going to press on your wrist." Then press three times on the exhale.
3. Now, again, speaking close to their ear, ask them about the different perceptual channels, and try to find where they are. Ask them: "Are you seeing something? Hearing? or Feeling in your body or emotions? Are you experiencing external or internal movement? Are you interested in relationship or in hanging out with God or in some other kind of spiritual place?" After each question, watch very carefully for feedback, and identify the main channels they are using.

4.   Find ways to work in those channels. Amplify each channel verbally for example by saying: "See that more," or "Listen to that," or "Yes, that's the feeling you are having." Rather than interpreting at this point, use blank statements, like: "Feel that," or "Wow! What a movement." Know that the person in coma rides your waves of energy, so bring your enthusiasm and energy to the work. Next begin using your hands near or on the person's body. Amplify seeing by touching around the eyes very gently. Amplify movement by inhibiting, supporting, or sculpting the movement. Amplify sound by working on the jaws or around the mouth, throat, and chest areas, as well as by making sounds with the person, and adding on a new sound here and there. Amplify feeling through body-work techniques such as massage, acupressure, rocking movements that come from Traeger body work, and so many other possible methods of amplification and bodywork. Amplify spiritual states by following the body's movements around the altered states, encouraging these with voice and hands; for example, if someone appears to be flying, help them have this experience in their arms, etc. You would know this by following their signals. Common signals that may indicate flying are eyes going way up, arms moving like a bird or moving up, and sometimes back arching, as if the person might be able to go into the yoga bridge posture. Amplify relationship through experimenting with contact and withdrawal—through putting your cheek close to theirs and watching for feedback.

5.   Keep working with the person until something significant shifts. It may be that they wake up, or that you see other evidence that something has changed, like tense muscles are now loose, or attempts to open the eyes have shifted into deep rest. You don't have to do it all in one session, just go for a significant change.

6.   If you are practicing with a partner, ask them to give you detailed constructive feedback around what worked and what didn't. Then change roles and repeat the exercise.

These basic steps have made up the bulk of the Coma Work I have done over the years. I stay very close to sensory grounded feedback, for example, noticing how, if I move the arms in this or that way, the person responds.

After I have worked repeatedly following the different signals in the body, my next steps with my client when I am working on them in coma will be to add on working with binary communication through yes and no signals, then I can ask questions and get specific information. Exercise 1.3 gives you practice in how to do this.

One of my next major directions is to help the person make new neural pathways, that is, to help them reestablish connections that are no longer functioning. I am acting like a temporary wire that connects two wires that were previously connected. We know that one of the

Exercise 1.3
Binary Communication (For Two People)

1. Go back into the coma state and start in the same way as before, with the hook up, by making a deep and strong connection with where they are.
2. Again, find and amplify channels for about 10 minutes.
3. Make connections between different channels and activities happening in the body and heighten the state of awareness of the person in coma.
4. Now try to find a signal that is consistent for yes and no questions. For example, have the person consistently raise their thumb to indicate yes and not raise it to indicate no. In coma, it often takes longer to respond to a command like "please raise your thumb for a yes" so patience is required. I often wait up to about two minutes for a response.
5. Once I get this basic communication established, I try to find out specific information by asking yes and no questions, and then I wait for yes or no feedback. Try guessing more into the person's experience, and look for feedback. This would involve asking questions about their process. For example: "Are you afraid?" Then pause and wait for feedback. If it's negative, continue asking questions substituting are you "Angry?" Pause. "Lonely?" . . . "Ecstatic?" . . . "Are you flying?" "Are you swimming in the ocean?" I might ask questions about their recovery like "Would you like to come out of coma?" If the answer is yes, I would say, "Would you like to come out today?" If not, I would keep asking times like in a week, or a month, or three months, six months, or a year. I might ask questions like "Would you want to come out more if you could do your art, or live in France, or climb mountains," or other specific kinds of directions I think this person might want to be going in their life.
6. I would then put together this information with the signal information I already have about the person and reexamine my ideas about what the person is doing in coma, and what could help them come back from the coma if they so desired. For example, I may decide that the person actually does seem really interested in coming out very quickly, so I may change my strategy from very slowly building up the person's fluidity in different channels, to really intervening dramatically to see how they might respond to my challenges to use their whole self to come to the surface and wake up.

problems with brain injuries is that different parts of the brain have difficulty communicating with each other. As a coma worker, I become something like the temporary communication channel to reconnect these parts. One time I was at a restaurant and a friend of my wife came in with her husband. We had a long talk. He had been in some kind of plane crash and his wife had sat at his side for months during his recovery. She didn't know what to do to pass the time, so she told him stories nonstop about these electricians who were in there rewiring him so everything would work. He had been an electrician. This man had a full and remarkable recovery after being given no chance of any kind of recovery. They were both sure that he had rewired himself with her assistance. I also discovered with my patients that if I help them to reconnect different activities in their bodies that they seem to develop more awareness in general, and more awareness specifically in connecting these body parts. For example, I see someone, perhaps named Sam, moving his neck and then he starts to move his leg, and I say to him: "That is Sam moving his neck and leg, and feeling the connection between that leg and neck." I might then also run my hand from Sam's neck down his arm and side of his body to his leg to help him feel that connection. When I have done this kind of work with students in my workshops, they report feeling that they come out of the exercise feeling more connected to themselves and in a higher state of alertness. I have had experiences with coma patients where they begin to put these parts together, and then more and more parts start to spontaneously line up, and suddenly they are making movements and sounds that they have never made before, or are coordinating different movements and sounds in new ways. For example, with Paul, I helped him connect his head movement with moving his arms and feet, and then suddenly he began to move his lips and his eyes went way up. I encouraged that and then made a statement about his legs, arms, lips, hips, eyes, everything opened more, and he began to look to me like he was having an ecstatic experience. Here is an exercise (Exercise 1.4) that allows you to experience what it feels like to have someone remind you of the way these connections work in your body when they are functioning properly.

It is important to have some sense of what some of the meanings are behind a coma, and to understand why comas "make sense" in some ways, in regard to the development of the person in the coma.

Here are a few exercises to help unfold these ideas. The first (Exercise 1.5) provides insight into why a person might be in coma in general, and the second exercise (Exercise 1.6) offers insight into why a person might stay in a coma.

Exercise 1.6 is meant to help you feel into the reality of someone in a long-term coma.

INTO THE SENTIENT REALMS

In the last exercise (Exercise 1.6), I mentioned going down and meditating to drop more into your center in order to relate more to your

Exercise 1.4
Reconnecting the Brain
(Two Person Exercises to Practice First with a Partner before a Coma Patient)

1. Connect three or four different things that are happening with your partner's body, and then say the person's name and what different things you notice them doing and how they are connected. For example, John's eyes are moving, his mouth moves, he takes a deep breath, and there is a sound happening in his throat. So I say to him: "That is John moving his eyes, his mouth, taking a deep breath, and making a sound, and all these parts are connected to each other." I then trace this connection with my hand so John not only hears me say the words several times, but he also feels my hand tracing the connection. This is the basic procedure: identify what you notice and then connect the parts.

2. I might then also guess into some pattern of signals, as if it is something from a dreamland. If the person tightens different body parts, I might say "is that a cat ready to pounce, or a door slamming shut?" If there is a growling sound, is that a bear present or thunder? Let yourself dream into their signals and watch for their feedback. For example, with a client that had many different parts of their body going up, guess into their rising or their flying. So again, the step here is to identify the signal and then guess into it by giving it some symbolic meaning.

3. After your initial guess, look for some kind of theme connecting these movements. Before you guess, take a minute to drop down into your own center and guess into something that might be even deeper, and name a kind of essence experience such as opening up, or being in light or in love, or something similar to that. It is easier to guess into something deep in someone else if you take a minute to meditate and center yourself first, even if you only close your eyes and take a few deep breaths, it helps to give feedback from a deeper part of yourself to the deeper part of the other person.

4. Continue to unfold this by saying something like: This is John. He is opening up at some very deep level; let that opening happen so John's deepest self can come forward. That is Sam closing his hand; his face is tightening, as Sam closes down, searching for safety. There is Sally making a fist, making a sound, looks like she is angry, and under that anger is power and energy.

5. If you are practicing this with someone not in coma, before you switch and let them practice on you, the person who pretended to be in coma should give their feedback. Were you close at all to their experience? Did you get to something dreamlike or essential that is part of their recent dreams or experiences, or something they are thinking about or working on?

Exercise 1.5
The Meaning of Being in and Staying in Coma (Inner Work)

1.   What kinds of inner and outer change do you need to make in your life that you feel you can't make or even look at or consider making? What are the deepest issues in your becoming yourself that those issues are connected to?

2.   Imagine that you could only make those changes if you could go away for a significant time to where you were separated from your ordinary reality. If you were in a coma that helped you get closer to these changes, what would you be like in this coma?

3.   Express somehow that feeling, that experience you would get close to, with a slight movement with one hand. What is that hand communicating? Keep exploring the slight movement until it explains itself to you.

4.   Now imagine you have come out of coma. How would you keep in contact with this part of you as you move through your daily life?

5.   If you could think of a psychological or daily practice that would help you stay close to this place of development, what would it be? Give it a name.

6.   Try doing your practice now and see how you feel differently.

Exercise 1.6
The Meaning of Long-Term Comas

1.   Imagine that you are in a long-term coma. What kinds of things would you want to hear someone say that would make you want to come out? What sounds or music would you want to hear? What would you want to see in your mind or on the outside? What kind of feelings would you want to experience in your body? What kind of emotions would help you come out? What would you need to experience in relationship that would cause you to want to come out? How about what world experiences would you need to influence you or to be able to influence from your coma state? What spiritual experiences do you long for or are you having that would help you come out?

2.   What kinds of experiences might make you not want to come out? Are there any experiences that you would feel strongly enough about that you might want to die to get away from?

client's deeper nature. To be able to reach our clients, we need to be able to go into these more sentient essence-like parts of ourselves. One of my main purposes in writing this book is to focus on how to develop your sentient nature to work with the client. By being able to go into our own sentient, essential places, we narrow the gap between ourselves and the person in coma. In one sense, the only difference between the more advanced person working with the person in coma and the person in coma is that the coma worker can go in and out of the state, and the person in coma is stuck in the state. I am always so touched by the experience I have when I have family members lie down and imagine that they are in coma. They talk about how relaxing it was and how interesting and how they didn't want to come back too quickly. The difficulty is not what happens in these states, it is learning how to get in and out of them. Being in an altered or extreme state can be exciting, restoring, and transformative, but being stuck in these states is a whole different experience. It might also be that the coma worker, by going in and out of the states, models something for the person in coma.

First, let's look at an exercise to learn how to drop into sentient realms. Then we will do another exercise that is specifically based on learning how to apply these methods to working on a coma. The first exercise (Exercise 1.7) comes from Drs. Arnold and Amy Mindell. If you are ever in the room with someone in a coma, try this exercise and you may suddenly know all kinds of new information about yourself, the person in coma, and the worlds that you both live in.

The purpose of this exercise is to give you an experience of the BIG YOU sense of your totality that goes beyond your limited thinking of who you are. The coma patient may be also, in their own way, trying to

Exercise 1.7
Into the Sentient Realms

1. Sit quietly and take a few breaths.
2. Close your eyes and let your mind become cloudy and unknowing. When your mind is empty, slowly open your eyes and notice whatever first catches your attention.
3. Notice what catches your attention and notice your feelings as you look at whatever it is that is flirting with you.
4. Shape-shift into the thing that caught your attention. For example, if you saw a picture of a river on the wall, let yourself become the river.
5. Now imagine that you could look back at yourself through the eyes of the river (or whatever caught your attention). What does the river see when it looks back at you?
6. Next, see if you can look at yourself and the river from the perspective of the BIG YOU, who sees the river and you as parts of the same whole. Take this as a momentary picture of the deeper you that is trying to manifest.
7. Imagine that you are this whole self. How might having access to your whole self help you with your struggles in some area of your life?

access this BIG YOU, and your being able to access it in yourself gives you more access to the world of coma patients.

When I want to move into the sentient realm, I use my eyes, hands, awareness in general, and my energy differently. Here is another exercise (Exercise 1.8) to get you more in touch with how to be in contact and work with the sentient level of awareness.

The purpose of this next exercise (Exercise 1.9) is to give you practice with learning how to use touch and do bodywork from this deep feeling place within yourself. The first step in moving into these more sentient-based, shamanic healing powers is learning how to believe in them and how to access them. This exercise can help you learn to believe in yourself. Two of the most important aspects of this Coma Work are to tell the client to believe in what they are experiencing, and coma workers need to take the same medicine and learn to trust their own powers of healing.

This is one of the most useful, powerful ways to do bodywork with a coma patient. Most of the time we touch each other while in an ordinary state of consciousness, such as my giving you a back rub while I am thinking about paying my bills. However, if I go into these deeper parts of myself, I will touch you in a very different way. When I did one of these exercises in a seminar, I demonstrated with my partner, Sage. I touched her hands from this essence place in myself. She said I had never, in 14 years of being together with her, touched her like that.

Exercise 1.8
Going Further into the Invisible

1. Imagine you could run a scan of your body with your body awareness.
2. Catch a body feeling that catches your attention, perhaps something that is surprising, something subtle, small, and not too scary.
3. Place your focus there. Feel it and try to amplify it a bit. It sometimes helps to breathe into that spot. Bring this feeling into movement and sound.
4. Now try to get to the essence of that feeling that is the first tendency or the seed of it, before it grew bigger and became that feeling in your body. One way to do this is to just feel the tendency to move *without* actually moving. Then begin to make very small, slow, sentient-like movements. Keep doing this until the deep feeling behind the movement reveals itself to you. You know you are at the sentient level when there is nothing against the experience you are having and you recognize and feel yourself embracing the experience. Let your mind formulate that and use it in any way you like. Express that essence in movement and sound, until you can name the un-named.
5. Let that experience come up to the level of words, and make some notes about what you learned about yourself in this exercise.

Exercise 1.9
Touching with Awake Hands
(Get Client's Permission Beforehand on Where It Is OK to Touch and Work)

1. Before you touch your client, let yourself take a few deep breaths. Scan first your own body and feel into where you connect to the deepest part of yourself. When you find that place in yourself, take a few breaths into that area and notice the feelings present there. Whenever touching your client, if you feel you lose contact with yourself or the client, go back to where you feel that deepest energy connection in yourself.

2. Now scan your client's body with your eyes and hands and notice where you feel their energy is somehow blocked. Notice a part that seems to want your attention or is drawing you to it in some way. Find a specific area that wants more attention. Follow the way to where your hands and eyes feel drawn to work. Let your hands feel into and follow what they sense. Watch carefully for feedback.

3. Close your eyes and feel and imagine and dream into that area you feel drawn to. Let a story emerge and report to your client what is happening and watch their feedback.

4. Take time to bring up all of the feelings that go along with the story, and notice how bringing them in affects your partner.

5. Find a way to bring some kind of resolution or healing to this story, that is, find resolutions for the client. State the resolutions. The healing process can be a co-creation. The two of you work together to find some healing path through these stories, based on the client's feedback. I would do this by making a resolution, then watching the client's feedback, and changing the resolution based on their feedback.

In summary, all of these different levels in Process Work are important to help the client to become more connected to themselves and their process. These exercises have two major purposes: to show you how to work with people in the realm of coma and to give the reader experiences in working and being in states that resemble coma to be a more compassionate and effective coma worker.

Chapter 2

The Myth of Vegetation: Mind-Body Beliefs and Coma Work

Chapter 2 places Process-oriented Coma Work within the context of recent mind-body theories, and it develops a new medical paradigm that goes beyond material causes and mind-body polarizations. This new paradigm is based on the idea of a creative and dynamic evolutionary process of co-shaping between mind and body and the meaningful flow of nature. It integrates not only Western allopathic medicine but also the philosophy and practice of both complementary medicine and spiritual healing and further includes findings from modern physics that show that matter and mind are complementary aspects of the same underlying reality.

INTRODUCTION

Pierre: The heart of our work, apart from the importance of all the practical steps, details of the hands-on work and relationship interactions, is a shift of mind set or paradigm. Coma Work requires us to reevaluate our understanding of health, healing, and process. In working with comatose people, their families, and care teams, this new view will be challenged at every step. Because of this we would like to go in depth with the details of the Process Work theory of health and process. It will help make all of the concrete applications easier to grasp.

In this chapter, we place our approach in the context of philosophical, cognitive, and Western medical theories and discuss their relevance for coma and the care of people who experience comatose states. We will further introduce Process-oriented Coma Work concepts within the context of recent mind-body theories and body psychotherapy.

These theories create the cultural context in which medicine and the care of people in comas is embedded. What people believe about the nature of their illness and disease affects both how they and their caregivers cope and deal with it. Knowing the cultural beliefs is relevant for understanding the various dynamics within medical systems and teams as well as within families and individuals who experience coma or having a loved one in coma. Raising awareness about these belief systems will hopefully allow you to better understand yourself and to better facilitate the relationship with everybody who might be involved in the care of someone in a vulnerable state such as coma or other conventionally nonresponsive states.

Our passion is to research and develop a new Process-oriented medical paradigm that goes beyond material causes and mind-body polarizations. This new paradigm believes in a dynamic and creative evolutionary process of co-creation between mind and body and the meaningful flow of nature. It includes allopathic medicine and also the findings from modern physics that show that body and mind are complementary aspects of the same reality. In a Process-oriented paradigm, healing occurs not only by addressing the material causes like putting a cast on a broken leg, but also by following the dreaming process of a symptom. You can take an aspirin to make your headache feel better, and if it feels like a pounding sensation you can also get into the pounding and discover the power of that pounding experience. From a holistic viewpoint the pounding sensation and the constriction and dilation of the blood vessels in the brain that may be the physical cause of the headache are both reflections of the deeper process of an unlived, life-affirming power.

PHILOSOPHICAL PRINCIPLES AND THE SURGE OF MODERN SCIENCE

There is a seemingly unbridgeable rift between an abstract world of ideas, hopes, beliefs, joys, and fears and a material world of cells, neurotransmitters, and hormones. How can mind, consciousness, self-awareness, a unified sense of identity, soul, and spirit come out of physical processes? Does the brain produce the mind, and if so, how? How much brain does it take to create the experience of mind? Is the mind really nothing more than sophisticated brain functions? If it is, how do we explain what happened between Erin and me? To answer these questions let us look at what philosophers and medical scientists have to say. For the sake of simplicity, we will for now differentiate only between two worlds and assume that the world of mental processes consists of a variety of experiences such as mind, consciousness, spirit, soul, psyche, and identity. We will later explore some definitions and develop a process-oriented paradigm.

In Europe the rise of modern science began in the Renaissance period. Before then the institutional Church's viewpoint was that God permeated all aspects of life and the body was the expression of God's work and plan and was therefore divine. Thus using the body for medical or anatomical research was perceived as a sacrilege. In the Renaissance period, thinkers and philosophers reoriented themselves toward Greek philosophical ideas and rediscovered a vision of man as a rational being. Later, Rene Descartes initiated a *dualistic* view of reality. He differentiated between thinking things and extended or material things. Life, he thought, was split in half: spirit or mind had no material foundation and it couldn't join matter or the body. One motive for Descartes to stress that matter was totally inert and insentient was the desire to use the human body for research. The distinction between mind and body allowed him to examine and dissect the body without offending the Church and his own spiritual beliefs. This separation between mind and body still permeates many of our beliefs today, though often not consciously.

This philosophical paradigm shift led to a medical revolution and an increasing understanding of the material and mechanical aspects of the body. By stressing the material aspects of the body, medicine initially neglected the mind. For many years the realm of mind and spirit was delegated to the Church or other spiritual institutions and thought of as not being a serious domain of scientific research. Later, with the advances in brain research, mind and spirit were viewed purely as a function of the brain. Many researchers have difficulties integrating the notion of a non-physical soul, spirit, or consciousness with the material aspects of the body. The idea of a separation between mind and body or spirit and soul and body leads to all sorts of riddles: Which parts of the physical world possess consciousness and which ones do not? Is the whole human body conscious or only the brain? How does consciousness attach to the brain and at what level of evolution does it enter the world? How does consciousness coexist with physical laws? The new thinking goes so far that nowadays most scientists believe that matter explains every aspect of reality. This totally materialistic view is replacing Descartes' dualistic separation between mind and body and scientific paradigms are now based on the idea that the mind is totally determined by the brain and has no nonmaterial existence.

However, both these philosophical principles about life and reality persist in today's Western cultures. The standard view, the one that many men and women in the street believe and many spiritual and theological views endorse, is usually dualism; that is, in addition to the physical or material world there is a separate mental or spiritual world. From a dualist viewpoint, an independent mental reality exists that is not part of the ordinary physical world. In opposition to dualism is materialism, which believes that the material world is all there is, and either consciousness has to be reduced to brain states or something absolutely physical, or else it doesn't really exist at all. So the big debate today is between dualism, which says that we live in two separate worlds, a mental world and a physical world, and materialism, which says no—it's all physical. Later we will explore the possibility of a third Process-oriented model, which is neither *dualistic nor materialistic* or both *dualistic and materialistic*.

Materialism is the foundation of current mainstream Western medical culture and practice and is the prevailing view among many professional experts like doctors, psychologists, philosophers, and neurobiologists. Materialism limits itself to the material aspects of life and marginalizes any other factors that generate or participate in the process of life. A medical science that is based on this materialistic assumption is supposed to be timeless, universal, and objective. From this perspective medicine sees reality as factual, objective, and "set in stone." Consciousness is based on a modern understanding of the human brain as a collection of brain cells that function in fundamental units or networks. The prevailing concept is that the brain works like a computer and consciousness mirrors a computational process. The favored theory is that conscious experience emerges at a critical threshold of complexity. Based on this theory, mental processes appear as a new biological property at a specific point of complexity in the evolution of life. Nevertheless, supporters of a science of purely materialistic and naturalistic beliefs, void of any metaphysical dimension, need to explain exactly how mental processes evolve from physical structures and what complexity is required to produce consciousness.

This model is also called the *biomedical model* and with its materialistic view of the body, it has contributed to huge technological progress in medicine. The unlimited access to hard facts has allowed the development of previously unimaginable therapeutic interventions. Because of these developments today, people survive severe injuries that only a few years ago would have caused certain death. If Descartes had not paved the road for medical discovery and progress, then Erin, the woman

I mentioned in the introduction, would almost certainly have died of her brain injuries. But her unique and unexpected reactions to my joining in with her experience cannot be explained by the existing materialist biomedical model. That experience challenged my medical beliefs and will hopefully lead us to a better understanding of the complex dynamics and processes that comatose people go through and to the development of a new paradigm.

As a result of this materialist orientation in medicine, most badly injured and comatose people are treated as if they are broken machines, and brain injured people who have severe brain damage are perceived as having no awareness or experience. In 1972, Jennet and Plum[1] first defined the clinical criteria for a Vegetative State of "wakefulness without awareness." People who suffered a severe brain injury, as a consequence of either a trauma or a lack of oxygen because of heart failure, would often wake up from coma into a state of recovered wakefulness during the day, but without any obvious signs of consciousness or awareness. The newly defined diagnosis of vegetative state was meant to describe this state and make sure that people understood their loved ones were not aware of their surroundings. This vegetative state was observed to be either a transitional state on the route to further recovery or could become chronic.

Subsequently, a Multi-Society Task Force[2] from various Western countries distinguished between a persistent vegetative state and a permanent vegetative state without chance of recovery. A permanent vegetative state was thought to be present after three months following a nontraumatic brain injury and twelve months after traumatic injury. A permanent categorization meant that the prognosis for patients in that state was very poor. However, some patients still slowly recover after many years and demonstrate transient signs of consciousness. Thus in 2002, the Aspen Neurobehavioral Conference Workgroup[3] from the United States published the definition and diagnostic criteria for a Minimally Conscious State. Patients in this minimally conscious state will show more than the purely reflex or automatic behavior that patients in a vegetative state show evidence of. They might track people with their eyes, respond to instructions to move a certain body part, and show other signs of basic consciousness.

A medical attitude that is based on the material attributes of life is static and focuses on individual disease states (persistent/permanent vegetative state, minimally conscious state) rather than on the life energies that move us and force us to adjust to the constant changes of our lives. There are currently approximately 35,000 Americans in a medically defined vegetative state and another 280,000 in a minimally conscious state. Unfortunately, most of these patients are treated as if they have no inner life and no experience of their environment. Most doctors believe that people like Erin are essentially "all gone," that although there is a human brain contained inside those cranial shells, something has gone away or is missing, something that holds the secrets of that person's soul. Many of us also believe that people in the final stages of Alzheimer's disease or in a vegetative state after brain injury are in essence all gone. The "I," soul, or spirit has either wholly or partly vanished, destroyed by the brain injury or the degenerative changes of the demented brain.

But to many people (ourselves included), this orientation is too limited and does not capture the fundamental nature of our being or our lives. In my experience with Erin, I had the feeling that there was no one home most of the time until unexpectedly she came out to connect with me in a unique and powerful way. This changed me so much that I now favor an attitude and orientation that values subjective experiences and the uncertainty of fluid processes. From this perspective, subjective features are as essential to reality as objective facts, and the ongoing organic changes and transformations of life are as relevant as individual disease states. The narrow focus on objective scientific knowledge has brought medicine a huge increase in effective treatments, but it has also become a problem because it misses the important relational and experiential aspects of human life, and it limits our expectations of what is possible.

From a materialist point of view, consciousness is very fragile and depends on physiological conditions that can be altered and annihilated by brain damage. Also, the permanent vegetative state is unquestionably a state in which patients lose their ability to communicate their conscious life in conventionally understandable ways. However, for many of us the source of conscious experience is the indivisible "I," which creates the unity of lived experience. This unifying process can't be explained in principle through matter only. Nobody has been able to explain how the brain creates a sense of unity and identity. In our view, conscious life itself is not limited to brain states.

Patients in states in which they cannot conventionally communicate about their inner experience need a new approach and a sensitivity that addresses their whole being. If consciousness emerges from matter or brain states then brain injuries will lead to consciousness injuries. Alternatively, if consciousness has an effect on matter, it must be separate from it. This materialist dilemma stems from a Newtonian view of cause and effect. In this book we represent a holistic or unifying new world view that transcends the polarization and holds the paradox by allowing mind and body to be two expressions of the same underlying process, which is functionally identical rather than separate. In this world both the subjective experience and the objective facts are true. We would like to propose a more subtle psychology and medicine that are based on awareness of both the everyday reality of limited time, space, and matter and a timeless dreaming reality.

Terri Schiavo's and her family's publicly debated struggle illustrates the current polarization between these different philosophical viewpoints and demonstrates the very concrete impact they have on people's lives and how they can influence decisions about life-altering treatments or their withdrawal.

DEFINITION OF CONSCIOUSNESS AND THE MIND-BODY PROBLEM

Definition of Consciousness

The definition of the term "consciousness" is difficult and laypeople and scientists use the term in many different ways. One dictionary definition is that consciousness is the awareness of one's surroundings, of one's situation, and of one's thoughts and feelings.[4] Similarly Solso[5] defines consciousness as the awareness of environmental (for example, sounds) and cognitive events (for example, memories, thoughts, feelings, and bodily sensations). Plum and Posner[6] define it as the state of full awareness of the self and of one's relationship to the environment. These definitions leave out the issue about the individual's ability to communicate about such awareness and the extent and/or form in which that communication is transmitted and received.

Another way is to define consciousness as a range of states of wakefulness and awareness in which one's ability to communicate with inner and outer worlds is preserved. Consciousness from this perspective is gradual on a continuum between wakefulness, sleep, and coma. This definition underlies the medical approach that denies any meaningful experience in coma. Additionally, consciousness is used to describe subjective experience. Consciousness then stands for the content of inner experience from one moment to the next. More globally, consciousness can be equaled with spirit/mind and used to describe the experience of human existence. It contains collective and individual values, hopes, and fears and defines our individual and collective identity. Consciousness has been used to describe a definite circumscribed process of awareness and communication of such awareness. It also stands for an ineffable sentient process, a world that seems to elude a materialist description.

These definitions are no doubt adequate for daily purposes. Nevertheless, they shed no light on the question of where this awareness is being registered. We can't currently measure consciousness; medical science has yet to develop a consciousness monitor. No technology is able to detect the physical signs of consciousness in a patient with any certainty. The newest technologies allow the monitoring of brain processing, but there is no consensus about how much processing or what type of processing qualifies as consciousness. There is no method yet available to clinically assess "internal awareness" in a patient who is otherwise unable to express awareness relative to external environmental stimuli. Clinicians are only able to *infer* the presence or absence of conscious experience through the observation of behavioral reactions to external stimuli. Nobody knows what exactly is to be measured. One example of this is when anesthesiologists struggle with surgical patients who experience some sort of consciousness while under general anesthesia. The phenomenon of consciousness does not have clearly defined boundaries, and the medical field has no established consensus as to what should count as the criteria for consciousness.

As we have seen, most scientists believe that the mind somehow *is* the brain, that matter and mind, brain and consciousness, are one thing. Consciousness for them is caused by the brain and a feature of the brain. Most believe that neuroscience will give us the answers to the mind-body problem. Science was able to explain the chemical and physical processes behind the burning of wood and it will in the future be able to give us the tools to understand the mind as part of the brain. Just as a medieval alchemist was confused about fire, current neuroscience has just not progressed far enough yet to be able to explain consciousness.

Others believe that consciousness is not physical, that it is another sort of thing altogether or that body and mind are a unity of which body and mind are each partial facets. They think consciousness is a fundamental entity in the universe, like mass, time, or space and that it penetrates the universe all the way down into the natural order of things. They bridge biology, neuroscience and psychology with quantum physics to understand consciousness as a fundamental aspect of the universe. They connect consciousness to physical concepts like quantum field, pilot wave function, vacuum energy, and Einstein's Æther and spiritual concepts like Qi, Tao, Prana, and God. We will develop this idea in more detail later.

So far, the problem of consciousness exists on two separate levels: Is the dilemma essentially a result of a false commitment to a materialist framework and therefore requires the recognition of an immaterial realm? Or does the mystery reside in our current lack of knowledge and limited understanding of the brain processes?

Some scientists argue that we as humans will never understand the nature of the process of how the brain generates consciousness.[7] And, most researchers agree that the mind-body problem and the definition of consciousness contain some "explanatory gap."[8] What is controversial is whether there is just a lack of knowledge and understanding or also a deeper basic lesson that needs to be drawn from it.

Mind-Body Problem

In our experience we seem to occupy two worlds: the world of the body and physical reality with its material and mechanistic properties, and the world of the mind with its mental or cognitive properties. One can also rephrase the mind-body problem to the question: Do you think that you *have* a body or that you *are* a body? Do you have a soul, spirit, or an indivisible "I" that somehow contains the unity of your experience and is independent of your body? Or do you think that your mind is an embodied part of a bigger, unifying whole?

We saw that many neuroscientists and philosophers have struggled with these issues at length. These are important issues with significant implications; whatever conclusions are drawn will have a big impact on how people are treated. If you are a materialist you will have the tendency to treat comatose patients as vegetating bodies void of any meaningful experience, which will hinder your ability to continue to perceive them as sentient beings. However, if you believe as we do that consciousness and the material body are complementary aspects of the same fundamental reality, you can open yourself to the idea that comatose people continue to have meaningful experiences despite their lack of being able to communicate them in a conventional way.

Descriptions of Mind-Body Interactions

Coma Work—the method we are proposing for working with people in outwardly unresponsive states of consciousness, because they don't communicate in conventional ways and we can't relate to them the way we are used to—is based on Arnold Mindell's Process-oriented Psychotherapy, which is part of the growing field of body psychotherapy. It also may be better viewed as "holistic psychotherapy" or "bodymind psychotherapy." Because the central way of relating and communicating is through verbal interaction, many of us feel at a loss when the verbal channel is blocked. Without verbal communication, regular psychotherapy is obsolete. In Coma Work we therefore focus on embodied relating using body psychotherapy methods that we developed in Chapter 1. In this section we will describe some of the "mechanics" of mind-body and body-mind interactions to better understand how body psychotherapy "works."

There are many figurative turns of phrase that we use and live by that describe the relationship between mind and body. In our Western culture, mind is described as a thing. We talk about the mind as a machine and as a fragile object. Examples are: "My mind just isn't functioning today," "I'm a little rusty today," or "His mind snapped." Other spoken images describe the impact that experiences have on the body: "She/He gives me a headache," "This event broke my back," or "This experience shattered him/her." We also generally assume that the conscious mind controls our voluntary functions and actions and takes it for granted in everyday life.

But exactly how the mind exercises its influence is not clear. There are four distinct ways one can conceptualize how body/brain and mind/consciousness might interact:

1. The body interacts with other physical substances and objects. This is the realm of conventional medicine and other body therapies. Consequently, the proper treatment is assumed to be some sort of physical intervention. If you over-exercise and develop muscle cramps, a physical massage will relieve the cramping, or if you suffer from migraine headaches in which brain vessel dilation causes pain, a chemical substance that counteracts the dilation will help.

2. Changes in your body, such as your brain chemistry, will cause mental and/or emotional disturbances. Current biomedical theories assume that changes in the levels of the neurotransmitter serotonin cause depression. Logically, this is the realm of biological psychiatry that then promotes psychoactive drugs to counter the effects of the brain's psychological disorders.

3. Mental and emotional processes cause mental problems. If you become depressed because of some losses in your life, you might seek some form of counseling. This is the realm of many forms of verbal psychotherapy that assume that psychological disorders can be alleviated by means of counseling interventions.

4. Mental processes cause physical problems. High loads of stress and/or emotional challenges can lead to diseases of the body such as stomach ulcers and high blood pressure. This is the realm of psychosomatic medicine. Consequently, under certain circumstances a physical disorder may require or benefit from a psychological intervention.

The conventional biomedical model limits its scope to the first two interactions and defers the third to psychotherapy. In the beginnings of the 20th century, Franz Alexander led the movement looking for the dynamic interrelation between mind and body. Around the same time both Sigmund Freud and Georg Groddeck pursued a deep interest in psychosomatic illnesses and researched the possibility of treating physical disorders through psychological processes. Together they initiated the field of psychosomatic medicine, which studies how mental processes cause physical problems. George L. Engel later developed the "biopsychosocial" medical model, a theory that expands mind-body theories to include social influences and believes that psychological and social phenomena have an effect on a wide range of bodily processes. It describes how mental and emotional states caused by social, cultural, and individual psychological processes are translated into neural, endocrine, and immune responses[9] of the body and in this way can contribute to, or even cause, disease. Both the psychosomatic and biopsychosocial model tried to overcome the dualistic division between mind and body.

In body psychotherapy, "the subject is neither the mind alone nor the body alone, nor even the two linked or in parallel—but the *body-mind*, a unity of which body and mind are each partial facets."[10] Coma and many other processes that alter our ability to relate and communicate force us to try to understand what we are, what our nature is, and what to make of the fact that we live as spiritual creatures in a universe full of mere material stuff. Do we believe that our consciousness is something other than a product of physical principles, or do we believe it is a byproduct of physiological process, or is there a third way? Over the years, medical doctors have researched and described a wide variety of mind-body interactions. They include studies of how guided imagery and biofeedback can be beneficial in relieving pain; studies of the placebo effect—how beliefs about a certain drug or intervention will impact the outcome or healing potential of that drug or intervention— studies of the negative effect of stress and trauma; and studies of meditation's efficacy in mitigating distress and increasing well-being. The theories that were drawn on to explain these interactions include both mechanistic and dualistic models.

In general, many medical models and practitioners omit the mind-body question by limiting their scope to the body. Others imply a dualistic approach or stand explicitly for a materialistic philosophy. I am constantly facing the dilemma and wondered many times if I rejected dualism would I have no other choice but to become a materialist. Then, dualism includes the possibility of an immortal part of ourselves and may ease some thoughts about death. To my understanding classical Newtonian physics doesn't allow for a third way, but quantum mechanics as we will see opens the door for a unifying theory of a *bodymind*.

For centuries doctors and healers have observed that difficult life circumstances change their patients' ability to stay healthy. Material troubles and/or the lack of access to sustaining resources were obvious factors that contributed to the weakening of the body's defenses. But they also observed that emotional challenges and traumatic experiences affected their patient's health. War veterans present with increased susceptibility to developing diseases like cancer, heart problems, and many others. Initially, most explained the increased health risks as a result of unhealthy behaviors. But then, veterans who lived healthy lifestyles became sick, too. To account for this, Hans Selye adapted within a mechanistic framework the notion of stress from engineering[11] to describe the body's ability to either adapt to or suffer from both material and emotional challenges. From this viewpoint the body's reactions to stress are determined by the interplay of several physiological systems (immune, neural, and endocrine). Recent scientific advances in these different fields have led to a clearer understanding of the connections among these systems, revealing possible mechanisms by which the body responds to environmental and social stress. Several modulators of stress and important variables in the link between the environment and the individual body have been described (for example, the hypothalamic-pituitary-adrenocortical axis [HPA] and the neurotransmitter serotonin[12]). In that way stress has been linked to depression, schizophrenia, suicidality, aggressive behavior, chronic pain, and many other stress-related physical diseases.

The latest biopsychosocial attempt to describe how stress mediates the disease causing effects on the body focuses on the body's ability to maintain stability during the course of change. If the daily hassles and chronic stressors are too challenging, the body will experience some wear and tear due to over-stimulation and get sick. The stresses that can break down our defense mechanisms are multiple. They can start when we are still in the womb and continue through infancy and adulthood. They include trauma and abuse as well as ongoing feelings of not being good enough and having low self-esteem.

Higher loads of stress can predict your risk of developing cardiovascular disease as well as a broad spectrum of other diseases (including circulatory, digestive, musculoskeletal, endocrine-nutritional-metabolic, nervous system, respiratory, and non-sexually transmitted infectious diseases).

Gary: The biomedical model is strong in explaining and identifying the stress factors, the stress physiology and the long-term pathological consequences of too much stress. In this model stress is seen as unhealthy and something that needs to be avoided. On the other hand, getting rid of stress may not work in today's world. In contrast a Process-oriented model believes that processing stress may be very useful to the person and good for their health. There is a difference between stress that we experience as being out of our control and that we feel victimized by and stress that we can learn to welcome as a challenge and opportunity for growth.

From a Process-oriented perspective, how stress is mediated or experienced is determined by the individual's process and his or her dreaming. For one person something is a challenge, exciting, energizing, fun, and healing; whereas for the next, the same outer factors may be debilitating to mind, body, and spirit. A pathological view of stress makes us feel like victims: knowing we live in a stressful world, we should be stressed out about stress! For example, many people come to me and say that after their physicals they were told they shouldn't have so much stress, which really stressed them out. But this is not the only possibility; for many of us stress can act like vitamins. A woman I just heard about took part in a Native American Sundance—a physically and emotionally intense ceremony. The long period of dancing and fasting could have been stressful to her system, but then she had a remarkable healing of her chronic pain. So although we have this biomedical theory that social issues and tensions create symptoms, I also have the experience that while working on social tensions can indeed be stressful, the processing of our social conflicts can also lead to remarkable well-being.

We don't know how people experience stress in coma. Is it stress? Is it a launching pad for altered states? Is stress irrelevant in such a detached state? Is there an amount of physical stress that can be useful and to what point?

Pierre: Nobody knows how a severely traumatized body or brain handles stress or ongoing emotional and psychological challenges. People in comas or persistent vegetative state have survived extraordinary harm and stress. They are dealing with ongoing physical, emotional, and spiritual trials. They need the support of a healing and care-taking community to foster their own self-healing capacity. The neglect that comes with an assumption that they lack consciousness or awareness unnecessarily amplifies the stress that some people in comas may already experience. Quite the opposite is needed. People in comas need all our sensitive and psychologically attuned interventions and support to accompany them on their recovery journey to relate to their internal awareness and consciousness, and thus to help them process their inner experience in a meaningful way.

Some researchers like Martin Seligman[13] have attempted to add a positive view on health and psychology to the predominant focus on the pathology and disease aspects of medicine. They have researched factors like resilience to stress and life challenges or what keeps us healthy despite the everyday harassment and ongoing stress. What they found out is that if we can assign meaning to what we have to live through and keep some even minimal sense of control over the life challenges, we have a better chance to stay healthy.

Our bodies respond to the way we experience life and our environment. Material problems, relationship troubles, and world events have a direct impact on our bodies through the way we are subjected to them. We say for example "You're a pain in the neck." Thus the world influences us and we affect the world around us. Mental imagery in music, sports, and in other creative arts is a crucial tool for all performers and is almost as effective as the actual physical enactment. What we imagine has a realness of its own. We can speak of a parallel and superimposed consciousness of the imaginary world and the consensually accepted real world. Our fantasies, brief thoughts and flirts, our dream images and feelings can all become embodied through the physiological reactions of our bodies. This also explains the self-healing capacity that we all possess and why psychotherapy works on the body and its symptoms as well as on the mind or psyche.

The theoretical problems posed by mind-body interactions can be illustrated by studies of imagery. Some researchers[14] have found that imagery can be an effective tool in exercising mental control over our own bodily states (for example, heart rate, blood pressure, etc.). The evidence that imagery can sometimes have direct physical effects suggests that the conventional, clear distinction between psychological reality and physical reality may not be quite so clear. As Kenneth Pelletier puts it:

Asthmatics sneeze at plastic flowers. People with a terminal illness stay alive until after a significant event, apparently willing themselves to live until a graduation ceremony, a birthday milestone, or a religious holiday. A bout of rage precipitates a sudden, fatal heart attack. Specially trained people can voluntarily control such "involuntary" bodily functions as the electrical activity of the brain, heart rate, bleeding, and even the body's response to infection. Mind and body are inextricably linked, and their second-by-second interaction exerts a profound influence upon health and illness, life and death. Attitudes, beliefs, and emotional states ranging from love and compassion to fear and anger can trigger chain reactions that affect blood chemistry, heart rate, and the activity of every cell and organ system in the body. All of that is now indisputable fact. However, there is still great debate over the extent to which the mind can influence the body and the precise nature of that linkage.[15]

Biomedical accounts usually relegate mind-body interactions to brain-body interactions. However this reduction of mental states to brain states or functions, in accordance with the view that mind and consciousness are nothing more than brain processes, still faces many difficulties. Exactly how imagery affects autonomic or immune system functioning has not been adequately scientifically explained and remains mysterious.

The limited biosociomedical view of disease hasn't found an answer to the mind-body problem. There is no understanding of how traumatic or stressful experiences or meditation and imagery are translated into physiology and biochemistry. The easy way out of the problem is to take a reductionist stance, make matter fundamental, and reduce mental states to brain states. Meanings, stories, and emotions are derivative: epiphenomena that ultimately reduce to matter. However, this still doesn't explain how a fantasy of a lemon stimulates one's saliva (just by reading these lines you as the reader may notice the change in your mouth); and how a conscious intent to lift a finger for typewriting makes that finger move also still remains a mystery; and so the question remains as to whether this is because science is not yet advanced enough or whether the mystery is an essential aspect of the process.

From an outside perspective the physical world appears closed. If one inspects the operation of the brain from the outside, one can trace the whole causal chain from sensory input to motor output without observing or needing any subjective experience. The brain machine works perfectly well without the need for any subjective experience to account for the neural activity that one can observe. To acknowledge mind-body interactions one needs to give an account of how the subjective experience and the body's reaction to one and the same event are related to each other. Further, we are not conscious of most of our own planning processes that precede a conscious action. We might have some awareness that relaxing music or imagery lowers our heart rate but we have no awareness about how it does it, so how could there be conscious control of such processing? In addition, Libet and other scientists have described that at least some voluntary acts are preceded by detectable neurological activity between 500 milliseconds and 10 seconds.[16,17] Thus, conscious experiences appear to come too late to have a causal effect.

These problems point to an impasse facing current efforts to solve the mind-body problem. How can experiences have a causal influence on a physical world that is causally closed or how can experiences affect processes that precede them? Both philosophical approaches (naturalist and dualist) have until now failed to answer the "how" questions. Faced with treating someone in coma or caring for a loved one in coma, these problems seem irrelevant. On a day-to-day level solving the question might not bring any advantages. But they are important when we want to explain how body-oriented psychological interventions can have an impact on someone's physical illness and coma.

Before exploring an alternative approach to the mind-body problem, let's explore how your own views influence your behaviors and the way you treat your body. Imagine or remember a body symptom or experience you had in the past or take a moment to focus on a body experience you currently have. Reflect on how you address the symptom or experience. What do you do to treat the symptom? Do you take medicine, go to a chiropractor, or do you choose to marginalize the experience? How do you explain your symptom or body experience? Do you associate it with a physical strain or any other cause?

Up to this point you probably used at least some materialist explanations. Now let's try to expand your approach. If you can, take a minute to relax and make yourself comfortable. Take a few minutes to focus on the subjective experience. How does the body area feel that contains your symptom or body experience? What are the sensations? Let the symptom explain itself to you. Explore some adjectives or images that describe the quality of the experience you are noticing. Use your imagination to discover your body and its expressions. Is it tender and in what way? Is it tense and what would best describe the tension? Give it some space and play with what you learn from your body.

While I was writing these pages I decided to take a break and walk to the coffee shop and continue to edit my manuscript there. I needed a change in surrounding and coffee seemed to be a welcome distraction. I walked quite rapidly across to the coffee shop and developed some slight exercise-induced asthma symptoms or tightness in my chest. I didn't have my inhaler with me but knew that coffee would relieve the symptom because of the Theophylline it contains, which is a natural bronchial relaxation agent. I also decided to explore my own subjective experience of the asthma. The tightness was slight and it felt like holding my attention to focusing on my inner states. It allowed me to go inward into a meditative space. I lost awareness of my surroundings and instead focused on going inside and taking a break. It actually helped me to take the break I was initially looking for. While I was meditating I also became aware of my fears and hesitations about coming out with my thoughts about coma. Being a scientifically trained medical doctor, it seems that I am venturing outside my field of expertise when I talk about philosophy and write about coma in a way that goes beyond conventional medical thinking. My "asthma" allowed me to stay in touch with a needed break from being outwardly focused and to go inside and process all the feelings and thoughts I had marginalized while writing these lines.

SYMMETRY AND CONSCIOUSNESS

To us . . . the only acceptable point of view appears to be the one that recognizes both sides of reality—the quantitative and the qualitative, the physical and the psychic—as compatible with each other, and which can embrace them simultaneously . . . It would be most satisfactory of all if physics and psyche (i.e., matter and mind) could be seen as complementary aspects of the same reality.[18]

In Greek mythology, if you were on the road to Athens, the center of all commerce, politics, and art, you had to pass by the ogre Procrustes and his Inn. In this Inn, Procrustes had only one size of bed. At night when you were asleep, Procrustes would come to your room and cut off any part of you that did not fit on his bed. If you were too short for his bed, he would stretch you until you fit. This myth represents what happens to all of us as we go through life trying to fit everyday expectations and goals. Parts of us get cut off or stretched so that we may meet certain expectations. As a community we have over time built a consensus about what reality is.[19] To be able to function as a community it makes sense that we need to agree on what reality is. We all need to follow certain conventions about the way we live together. Driving on the same side of the road and the reality of a red light as a signal for us to stop is important. If we didn't agree, chaos and injuries would ensue from some stopping and others not. This consensus reality is an important reality but not the only one. To fit into everyday reality some of us disassociate ourselves from the parts that are less consensual, more oriented toward creativity, dreams, and spirituality. Being diagnosed with an illness challenges many consensus reality views and values. This process may transform our identity and reconnect us with the forgotten parts. A holistic healing integrates both the consensus reality perspectives and the creative process of what we call dreaming.

Albert Einstein said: "Reality is merely an illusion, although a very persistent one." His relativity theory gives unusual answers to the question, what is reality? He described how the mass of an object depends on its speed relative to another object and so does its length. Since objects in the real world are always moving at slightly different speeds from one instant of time to the next, relative to one another, reality is only relative and has a brief lifetime! If we contemplate the relativity of our agreed upon reality we open ourselves to our inner diversity and the diversity of the world and the communities around us.

The physicist Wolfgang Pauli worked closely with the psychologist C.G. Jung. Before his untimely death from throat cancer in 1958, Pauli was passionately interested in how psychology and physics (mind and matter) fit together. In his quantum mechanistic approach he reconciles the two worlds of mind and matter and explains how conscious experiences can have an effect on the physical world. Other researchers since then claim that there is one "mental life" but two ways of knowing it: knowledge from our subjective experience and from the outside observed knowledge. Objective and subjective manifestations of our experiences are different complementary aspects of the same experience. Mind and matter are two expressions of a more primal quality or implicate order, as physicist David Bohm[20] portrayed it. Once consciousness or observation occurs, the "quantum wave function" collapses into subjective and objective reality. Physics' most modern understanding of the physical world suggests that there may be an ineffable realm, a mystical realm, an "imaginal" realm, out of which the physical world pops and/or comes into existence.

In quantum physics elemental particles behave either as waves or as particles. The quantum physicist's wave equation describes the probability of a particle having wavelike and particle-like characteristics. Which aspect of matter appears, wave or particle, depends on the decision of the observer. But as Arnold Mindell states: "We must remember that both wave and particle are consensus reality descriptions of an invisible world. Both descriptions together are considered complementary; both consensus reality terms are needed to approximate the measurable qualities and quantities of matter."[21] For physicists the wave function is considered to be the most fundamental description of matter. In its physical equation the wave function ends up to be a complex number that has both real and imaginary aspects and cannot be measured directly. This more fundamental imaginal realm is the ultimate Unreality that manifests itself to us in both physical and mental ways, but is itself more basic than either. Wilber[22] claims that the non-dual aspect of reality can only be experienced from a non-dual heightened state of awareness (for example, through contemplative practices and meditation). Mindell suggests that for the most part we marginalize the imaginary realm and orient all our experiences to consensus reality. "We look only for the most probable meaning of something . . . Metaphorically speaking, looking only at the real value of an experience gives us answers in reality, but ignores the sentient dreamlike experience and process of reflection behind reality . . . Consensus reality is like a tree with roots in the non-consensus or sentient realm."[23]

This sentient or imaginal realm is at the core of mythology and spirituality. It can also be experienced in subtle tendencies and dreamlike processes that one subliminally senses. According to Mindell, consciousness is based on sentient non-consensual tendencies reflecting on one another. For him, in analogy to the wave function and Bohm's implicate order, the sentient realm underlies and structures all of manifest reality.

CONSEQUENCES FOR A PROCESS THEORY OF MEDICINE

The medical world is in transition and at a crossroads. The 19th and 20th centuries saw the establishment of scientific medicine based on the view that human health is fundamentally biological. One the one hand, this deep biochemical familiarity with the human body along with nanotechnological engineering advances will, in the 21st century, set the base for an increasingly sophisticated molecular and technological medicine. Superspecialized and automated procedures that produce better treatment results, such as the surgical fixing of hernias[24] or colonoscopies, will no longer require the extensive training that medical doctors currently receive. Thus, many facets of medicine originally assigned to doctors could, and might soon, be done by machines, medical engineers, or expert systems and computer algorithms.

On the other hand, noncompliance, the lack of adherence to medical treatment, difficulties encountered in chronic symptom management, the issue of health disparities based on social strata, the problems of medical malpractice and litigation, as well as rising health care costs, all point to unsolved problems that can't be solved by the technological advances in medicine. The materialist biomedical model of medicine treats the body as if it were a machine that can be understood in terms of its parts. This model studies the body's elementary particles, so to speak, its atoms, molecules, and organs, the bits and pieces that make up the cells and the body. In today's medicine you are either sick or well. You have a body or a psychological problem which may be hereditary, or caused by stress or carcinogens, by too much fat or not enough vitamins. Social science expands the biological view of health to incorporate interpersonal, social, and cultural dimensions, so physiologic states become a metaphor for social and cultural processes, which are intrinsically entangled with relational and community aspects and call for a different sort of therapeutic model.

Diversity awareness, conflict facilitation, process and systems psychology, and cognitive and behavioral approaches are required to address these aspects of medicine that can't be replaced by machines or technical engineers. Nevertheless, the biopsychosocial model requires mental or psychosocial events to cross back over the mind/brain barrier and then influence the body via neural, immune, and endocrine pathways. It remains stuck in a dualist or materialist philosophy and fails to answer how experiences have a causal effect on a physical world.[25]

A Process-oriented or *non-dualistic non-materialistic* model of medicine and illness sees body experiences as not only local, physical difficulties, but also as processes that relate to the sentient or imaginal realm and includes both the biomedical and biopsychosocial approaches. The physical aspects and the subjective meanings of our experiences are complementary and different aspects of a sentient process. Sickness is a meaningful process that requires both our attention to find a cure as well as some processing to explore its meaning. The sentient realm encompasses the mechanical organization of the body and the subjectivity of the whole person. The philosopher of consciousness David Chalmers says: ". . . experience may arise from the physical, but is not entailed by the physical."[26] Consequently, experience or subjectivity is as fundamental as physicality—they both have their roots in the wave function of reality. Clinicians using a non-dual non-material model see the multidimensional nature of disease and approach clinical work from multiple complimentary observer positions.

Some physicists and astrophysicists[27,28] have a view of life that gives meaning and direction to evolution and its self-regulating creativity (for example, consciousness). Their metaphysical and teleological conceptualization of life that opposes *entropy*[29] and gives meaning and direction to evolution survives despite the dominance of materialism and scientism. In physics, Newton determined the forces controlling the fate of objects and saw them as lifeless. Leibniz disagreed and insisted on an inner force, the "vis viva," as the mover of matter, for only matter can move matter, and the spirit or energy that is able to move it is necessarily part of it. History has, for a certain time, decided in favor of Newton. On the other hand, Einstein's relativity theory ($E=mc^2$) asserts that every material object has an energy that is inherent within it. But as Mindell observes: "Newton's idea of lifeless matter still prevails in science, since energy is defined mechanically. Yet Leibniz's 'vis viva' hovers in the background, behind the new tendency of scientists on the cutting edge of physics who are exploring where consciousness enters matter."[30]

With the rise of genetics and evolution, vitalist ideas disappeared almost completely except within some departments of theoretical physics. Modern molecular biology ascribes life to an emergent property of biochemical processes and so any vitalistic life force or energy field is deemed unnecessary and unacceptable. Nonetheless, their functional descriptions still fail to capture the organizing principle present in living systems and consciousness, the kind of inherent wisdom that fuses together amino and ribonucleic acids into proteins, molecules, and organisms. New concepts of quantum theory are now being drawn on to explain basic intercellular and intermolecular dynamics and to revise our understanding of our physical bodies.

In a non-dual non-material medicine, the physical expression of disease is only one dimension. Mind and meaning are embodied in flesh. Body and mind are two complementary expressions of a basic embodied reality. The somatic language of the body conveys meaning for the individual, for his or her environment, and for the world at large. The meanings that emerge from the physicality of our bodies are complementary to psychological meanings. A clinician of non-dual medicine or psychology—from a non-dual non-material perspective the differentiation between medicine and psychology makes less sense—will attend to the many levels in which meanings or stories are communicated through illness and other life disturbances.

Embodied meaning is passed through specific personal experience, arises in the context of community and cultures, and is passed through generations. What is needed is a willingness to observe the unitary reality from multiple observer positions and to recognize that mind and body are fundamentally psychophysical. This allows us to make sense of the mind-body interactions we observe in clinical practice and everyday life.

Physical, emotional, and spiritual health is a privilege that we often take for granted. Most of us only recognize that privilege in hindsight once our health or the health of a friend or family member is challenged. At that time, many of us feel that our sense of stability and peace of mind is threatened. With physical and mental illness comes a questioning of our everyday identity and our goal and purpose in life. Some of us will be forced to reorient ourselves, face issues of loss and grief, and search for new meanings.

Of course there is nothing "good" about illness and no one living in even moderately good health wants to imagine ceasing to be the person they enjoy being. Nevertheless, confrontation with illness can initiate some growth opportunities and personal powers. Illness can be excruciatingly painful and difficult, and we all hope to be spared some of its pain. But at the same time, individuals confronted with health challenges often achieve deep and meaningful levels of psychological awareness. All of us would like our bodies and minds to allow us to live a normal life and to give us some minimal degree of comfort or absence of pain. Nobody looks forward to being ill and coma in particular is an extreme process and obviously challenging to come to terms with both for the loved ones and the person in coma. Presuming that there is some meaning to the experience is at best audacious. However, as Erin showed me, there is much more to her experience than we are used to perceiving. According to the existing biomedical model, she wasn't supposed to be able to show any emotional reaction or have any inner experience at all, but she did.

Medical progress has allowed us to keep people's bodies alive. However, we still lack knowledge in regard to understanding consciousness or to truly fathom what people go through when they face these life altering processes in coma and so-called vegetative states. Now new research is discovering evidence of consciousness in people who were deemed to have no inner experience at all.[31] We are starting to realize that people in these assumedly vegetative states are able to hear and understand instructions, retrieve a memory of a sport activity, including the concepts of what is involved in that activity, and keep their mind focused on that activity long enough for it to light up in a brain scan! In other words they are still having meaningful experiences and are able to relate to the external world as well as to their own inner world.

In her book, *One Unknown*, Gill Hicks,[32] who survived the London Underground bomb attack of 2005, describes how although she was moving in and out of consciousness and was unable to communicate verbally with her rescuers, she held on to the hand of one of them and could feel him willing her to live and, as she puts it, "sharing some of his life force with her." Later someone else noticed her eyes flickering and used blinking as a way to spell out her name. She describes her relief at knowing that now they would be able to contact her husband Joe, which helped her hold on and keep living. Staying related to people in these extreme states is so important and can make a difference between life and death.

Materialistic philosophical assumptions have prevented us from recognizing the lived experience of coma and from developing treatment methods that value these experiences. As medical doctors we are exceptional in treating the bodies and their malfunctions, but the mind stays elusive, especially when its manifestation goes beyond the scope of conventional communication. Thinking about philosophy and its implications is important if we want to open ourselves to new worlds of experiences. If you think back to the short inner work exercise you might appreciate both a materialistic approach and a non-dualistic method that gives value to the subjective realm. Using both ways of experiencing the world, the materialist angle and the subjective angle, allows us to find new ways to relate to people in various altered or comatose states as well as to treat their bodies in the best way possible.

Chapter 3

The Myth of Health and Normality

In this chapter, we examine mainstream medical ideas about health and healing that emphasize the re-establishment of ordinary states of consciousness, such as returning the patient to "being just like before the coma." We compare and contrast this with a Process-oriented approach to healing that expands our concepts of health and normality to include the wide diversity of our lived experiences. We discuss the biomedical view that is based on pathology and add the concepts of process, fostering self-healing, and meaning.

We also explain how to integrate mainstream medicine and Process-oriented Psychology to create a holistic approach. For example, using Process Work with a woman with fibromyalgia, we explored this woman athlete's constant pain in trigger points, point by point. Each point contained not only disease, but also incredible memories and dream-like experiences, from her hurtful mother in her arm pain to Achilles' strength and vulnerability in her Achilles' tendons. As we processed each point, her pain transformed into healing, release, energy, and transformation, until she was diagnosed as free of fibromyalgia.

WHAT IS HEALTH?

Pierre: To fully understand the shift in mindset, we need to think about health and healing. In Process Work we believe that health is a fluid subjective experience in the same way that illness is. We believe that there is a continuum of experiences that individual people, groups and cultures frame as being part of good health or disease. Health is not an achievable state that is clearly defined; it is rather a process that includes and is shaped by individual and cultural beliefs and values. Health does not exist without illness. And then, health and sickness are consensus reality concepts. Being healthy or sick are polarities that we experience in everyday reality. On another level, sickness and body symptoms are part of nature. They are processes that are part of the wholeness of life and its multiple manifestations. Thus, on a dreaming and sentient level, people are not sick and do not need healing. But when people have body symptoms, they feel something is wrong or they are in pain and the consensus reality aspects of their body symptoms need to be addressed. As experiences, body symptoms include a psychological dimension. Both health and illness have meaning and are part of a teleological and developmental process. To gain a better understanding of what wants to happen, we use the body experience as our guide. We take very seriously every detail of what people say and how they describe their experience, and we help them understand its meaning in their current context. If the experience feels like a pressure, we help them identify where they need more or less pressure in their life. As part of the experiential nature of health and illness, Process Work integrates all conventional and complementary medical aspects of health and illness: the assessments, diagnosis, treatments, relationship dynamics with health care providers, social and cultural issues, etc.

Let me now discuss other peoples' views and how they relate to Process Work ideas, concepts, and thoughts.

Hannah Arendt said that health as a word or concept is "something like a frozen thought which thinking must unfreeze."[1] In everyday language we take the meaning of the word *health* for granted. When we speak about health we assume a tacit understanding and general consensus about the notion of health. For instance, most people will agree that smoking is in general bad for your health. On second thought, however, the hidden difficulties of defining the concept of health become apparent.

For some of us, health is a core value of life and closely related to our general sense of well-being; for others, health is less central. Obviously, most people's preferred approach toward illness, after getting sick and suffering, is to get treatment and get through treatment to restore their health. Most doctors and health professionals will encourage this outlook and motivate behaviors that will restitute health and rehabilitate disability. This approach makes disease an enemy and to cure and overcome the disease you are supposed to conquer that enemy. Both patients and doctors team up to defeat illness, old age, disability, and ultimately death. An enemy is something we separate ourselves from, which is outside of ourselves, foreign, with a language that we don't understand, a process that we don't identify with.

Obviously, nobody likes to be sick and in pain, and to fight disease makes a lot of sense. But what happens with the unlucky ones who become chronically ill or who become severely injured or disabled? And what of our elders whose health slowly deteriorates and whose bodies become frail and weak? Marginalizing illness, old age, and death only works for some people and for a limited time. It is everybody's fate to have to embrace the enemy at one time or another whether we want to or not. Is there another way of relating to disease and pending death? Is it possible to embrace the process of illness and befriend the enemy? Most of us won't be able to do that most of the time and maybe we shouldn't. Embracing what causes pain and suffering is challenging and fighting it makes sense. When we feel sick or struggle with body pain we often feel victimized, and fighting back is an attempt to regain power and control. That is obviously a good thing and all of us need support for that. But is illness really only an enemy or are there things we can learn from this difficult process? How can we find meaning in illness? Can we both fight *and* open ourselves up to learning and using the challenge of illness to learn and grow? What would it entail to do both? These are the questions we will explore throughout this chapter.

"ARCHETYPE OF THE INVALID"

Guggenbühl-Craig speaks of a basic phenomenon of life that defies all healing efforts. He calls it the "archetype of the invalid."[2] Deficiencies, functional impairments, and symptoms are always part of ourselves. He regards health and invalidity as complementary archetypal fantasies and reproves a concept of wholeness that is one-sidedly identified with health. He argues that the prevailing idea that health is wholeness in mind and body ignores the processes of disease and invalidity that are within each of us. Splitting health from illness leads to a one-sided focus on health and wholeness and to negative stereotyping of people with symptoms. And, as we will see, this also leads to the body becoming a symbolic field for the reproduction of mainstream biomedical and *allopathic*[3] values. In Guggenbühl-Craig's opinion, the body may also become a site for resistance to, and transformation of, those systems of meanings. Sickness may be an unconscious expression of a struggle to resist and defend ourselves from the one-sided moralistic call for total good health. The ambition to heal everyone and everything forces a counteraction that resists the expectations of wholeness and good health. In this way the concept of health begins to feel oppressive, and we counterbalance it with seemingly irrational unhealthy behaviors.

The one-sided centrality of "good" health discriminates against ill and disabled people and those whose inner states and experiences are less strong and resilient. It also contributes to the isolation of individuals and families who experience health challenges, disability, and unusual states of consciousness. The focus on health and the emphasis of re-establishing ordinary states of consciousness, for example, rehabilitating the patient into "being just like before the coma" denies the validity of the lived illness, coma, or altered state experience. This one-sidedness plays a role in an unrealistic ambition and orientation in medicine to restore health no matter what, that oppresses everybody in it. Guggenbühl-Craig's "archetype of the invalid" stresses sickness as a basic phenomenon of life that often defies all healing efforts and has the potential to guide us all toward our ultimate destiny.

This is obviously controversial and will elicit many feelings and reactions. In Process Work we recognize the value of the tension between the opposites of health and illness and the dialogue it creates in us individually and in groups and communities. We see these polarities as aspects of our growth and learning as individuals but also as families and cultures.

UNCERTAINTY AND THE ROLE OF THE EXPERT

Illness and disease provoke fear and uncertainty. They throw us off balance and out of our ordinary lives. We are forced to confront our boundaries, limitations, and vulnerability. To avoid these difficult feelings we often look for an expert to whom we assign the task of doing everything in their power to restore our health. Doctors and other health professionals may both opt into, and suffer from, that delegated pressure to alleviate pain and suffering by all means possible. As patients we expect the experts to know exactly what to do and not to make any mistakes. We want clear answers, assurance, and certainty. Paradoxically illness and the uncertainty of not knowing can be relieving and refreshing and balances the pressures, ambitions, and expectations of the expert in all of us. Many people who have faced serious illness say they have gained from the experience. They say it helped them prioritize values and relationships and focus on what was important to them. I also believe it can be a powerful connector and makes us all more humane. It forces us to relate to our feelings and emotions and opens us to aspects of life that aren't yet controllable and solvable.

Because of their focus on health and expertise, current medical views tend to overestimate the importance of objectifiable cause-and-effect relations. In doing so, they disavow the influences of psychology, dreams, and non-local field effects. From our Process-oriented perspective, best medical practice combines scientific and technical mastery with the art of relationship improvisation and embraces uncertainty, uniqueness, and diverse value systems.

THE ROLE OF BELIEFS

From a Process Work perspective, beliefs are an intrinsic part of our experience and they have a strong influence on how we treat our bodies, how we think about health and coma, and how we relate to structures and systems that help us on our journey through health and disease. Beliefs are powerful and infectious. They are the building blocks of our cultures. They shape our thoughts and actions, and our relationships and community efforts. They are non-local in the sense of being shared by individuals, communities, and whole cultures. They form the philosophies and paradigms that inform our thinking and attitudes toward life, social interactions, and life-style choices. They create the field we live in and guide the roles that represent the polarities of the field. In an ongoing subliminal process of consensus building, they shape what we experience as reality, true and false, right and wrong. They are externally represented through the media and religious and scientific institutions, and we also experience them through internalized representations of our parents, teachers, and peers. They are good and bad medicine, placebo and nocebo. In health they shape our hopes and despairs and organize our physiologies.[4]

In the 1970s, breast cancer was believed to be deadly and many women died shortly after their initial diagnosis. Breast cancer is now much more treatable and the change in attitude toward breast cancer has added to the reduction of its mortality. Beliefs about consciousness also influence our efforts to rehabilitate severely brain injured people. Beliefs about brain plasticity, or the lack thereof, cause brain injured people to be neglected and marginalized. New treatments give us hope and change our beliefs and survival rates. Thus beliefs about the aging and injured brain determine the course of our loved ones recovery from stroke, Alzheimer's, and brain injury.

In his book *Man's Search for Meaning*,[5] Viktor Frankl, a Jewish psychiatrist and Holocaust survivor of the Nazi prison camps of Theresienstadt, Auschwitz, and Tuerkheim, found that if you had a goal then your chances of survival improved. He came to the crucial conclusion that if you have a goal and can find some meaning even in the most painful, absurd, and dehumanized situation, then you can develop inner powers and resources that give you a better chance of overcoming the challenges you face. To maintain his own feeling of meaning and purpose, Frankl imagined delivering lectures to his students and in his mind wrote the books he later published. He found that life is *teleological*; it is goal-oriented and directed toward a final result.

The United States lost more prisoners of war in the Korean War than in any other war. The casualty rate was about 40 percent. The North Korean and Chinese Communists used elaborate methods of indoctrination, which took away hope from the captives. Both in Nazi prison camps and in Korean or Chinese internment camps, prisoners who lost hope crawled into a corner or into their bunk beds, pulled a blanket over their heads and quit living within 48 hours; some died over night from no apparent physical cause. In many cultures individuals may be punished by a collective process of social expulsion or ostracism, a fate often practically equivalent to death. These examples demonstrate that hope and the belief in a meaningful existence is a central life force. When they are taken away it can be deadly. Medical attitudes and beliefs co-create the experience of illness and the course or outcome of an illness. In my view they have a relevant impact on the chance of recovery from coma and vegetative states.

Aaron Antonovsky,[6] an Israeli sociologist, studied hope in a different context. He studied women who had survived both the Holocaust and the following displacement and immigration to Israel, major life stressors that would normally result in impaired health. In his research he discovered a subgroup of women who seemed to have extraordinary resilience in facing these major life challenges. A characteristic of these women was that they had been able to keep a sense that their life path was somehow predictable and explicable, that they had the resources to manage the challenges, and that the life demands were worthy of investment and engagement. Antonovsky termed this psychological and spiritual power *sense of coherence*. According to Antonovsky, if a person believes there is no reason to persist and survive and confront challenges, and if he or she has no sense of meaning and direction, then he or she will lose the motivation to strive and live. In his research he demonstrated that a strong sense of coherence predicts positive health outcomes.

To conclude: if you have no supportive relationships, have no hope, goal, or sense of direction and meaning, you get sick and die. Love, hope, and meaning are excellent medicine. All medical treatment and care of a person in coma must include hope and love. Without it the chances of recovery are slim.

NEUROPLASTICITY

A specifically relevant belief in coma care is about the brain's ability to adapt, regenerate, and heal. For many years mainstream medicine believed that the brain could not change and that many neurological and psychiatric problems were "hardwired" in an unchangeable brain. The adult brain was not thought to be able to grow new nerve cells. This has changed in recent years with the discovery that the brain is much more plastic than previously thought. One of the origins of current interest in brain plasticity and brain rehabilitation is the story of the dramatic recovery of Pedro, the father of famous brain researcher Paul Bach-y-Rita.[7] In 1959, Pedro, age 65, experienced a stroke that left him severely disabled, unable to move or take care of himself. The family was told that their father had no hope for recovery and that there would be no benefit from extended rehabilitative treatment. George, Paul's brother, knew nothing about rehabilitation, but he simply didn't believe what he was told. He took his father home to Mexico and over one year taught him to walk, speak, and lead a normal life. Pedro resumed his full-time teaching at City College in New York, went mountain climbing and traveling, and lived for seven more years. After Pedro died from a heart attack, Paul asked a colleague to perform an autopsy. The autopsy revealed that Pedro's extensive brain lesions had not healed but that his brain had totally reorganized itself through the work he had done with George. This led to the emergence of the research in neuroplasticity and the belief in the brain's ability to re-organize itself.

Here is another fascinating story that resulted from Paul Bach-y-Rita's research. Cheryl, one of Paul's recent patients, had damage to her vestibular apparatus, the sensory organ for her balance system. A course of antibiotics she was given for a postoperative infection had poisoned her inner ear and upset her balance system to the point where Cheryl up to this point constantly feels as if she is falling. She is unable to stand or walk and even when she has fallen she continues to feel as if she is falling. By conventional medical criteria, Cheryl's situation is hopeless. But Paul's team is challenging that. They have developed a machine that replaces the balance system by transmitting information about Cheryl's body movements and accelerations to her tongue. When Cheryl bends forward small electrodes send little electric shocks to the front of her tongue and inform her that she is bending forward. With the help of the machine Cheryl has relearned to sense her body's motions in space and has slowly acquired the ability to stand and walk again. The most exciting aspect of the experiment, however, is that over time Cheryl's brain has also somehow learned to rewire itself so that Cheryl can now dance and has returned to normal functioning even without the machine.

In one particularly relevant study, Laureys, Boly, and Maquet[8] observed partial functional restoration of neural connections in patients who recovered from persistent vegetative states. They observed that long-distance rewiring of nerves is possible and is related to the new growth of neurons. They concluded that "chronically unconscious or minimally conscious patients present unique problems for diagnosis, prognosis, treatment, and everyday management. They are vulnerable to being denied potentially life-saving therapy if clinical research remains solely focused on the acute stage of the disease."[9] They state that "the residual cerebral plasticity in chronic disorders of consciousness has been largely overlooked by the medical community and deserves further study."[10] Collectively, the findings of this and many similar studies support neuroplasticity in both brain structure and function following severe injuries. Unfortunately, despite these findings, many doctors still believe that the adult human brain cannot change, especially when it has been severely injured.

The idea that the brain changes its structure and function all the time through stimulation and learning revolutionizes classical thinking in neuroscience. It has implications for our understanding of how relationships, addictions, culture, and psychotherapy change our brains. It brings hope for people with sensory, cognitive, and emotional impairments due to schizophrenia, autism, deafness, blindness, aging, learning disability, as well as brain injury and coma.

Current studies of neuroplasticity[11] show that if neural circuits receive a great deal of traffic, they will grow. If they receive little stimulation, they will remain the same or shrink. The brain adheres to a "use it or lose it" principle. If you don't use a certain path way or function, the neural or synaptic connections will become weaker. The amount of traffic our brain circuits receive depends mainly on our attention and motivation. This is significant for people in comas. In the initial stages people's attentions were turned inward without any signs of outward awareness. However, after a certain amount of time, most coma patients will reorient their attention outward by opening their eyes and re-engaging in a cycle of more awake states and sleeping states. The main problem is that there is a communication barrier between the comatose person's experience and us as outside helpers. This has led conventional medicine to call these states vegetative and equate them with lack of consciousness and experience.

The communication barriers and the beliefs associated with them have led to a lack of motivation in the helper as well as from the person in coma. This deficit in attention and attuned stimulation results in hopelessness and depression and in the development of secondary iatrogenic (medically induced) physical atrophy of brain structures. René Spitz[12] and John Bowlby,[13] two pioneering European psychoanalysts, showed that institutionalized infants failed to thrive and developed stress-related psychosomatic damages. Our failure to stimulate and communicate with people in comas has potentially very similar effects. The experience of neglect that people in comas have often results in "hospitalism," a condition of wasting away while in a hospital. Lack of stimulation and support is also stressful for them and increases their chances of sustaining further physiological damage due to the negative effects of stress hormones.

Neuroplasticity is thus both a blessing and a curse. It is the reason for being hopeful about recovery and the motivation for long-term specialized rehabilitation treatments. It can also be a problem in terms of the comatose person's reinforced learned hopelessness or helplessness and the isolation that results from our lack of understanding of these remote states of consciousness. Isolation, depression, and hopelessness result in brain changes. They create secondary damage on top of the initial injury. As medical providers and coma workers we need to help counteract and prevent these harmful changes. Hope and the belief in the brain's positive adaptability and ability to regenerate are our best medicines.

When people wake up from these states, a block often remains and most won't be able to recall or recount their coma experiences. However, some do and have told their stories. Many have spoken about the importance of their helpers' attitudes, how they felt either connected and supported or pushed away, which led them to recoil into a safe place inside themselves. To quote one such story: "As far as being aware, I remember much of what was going on around me during the coma. My surroundings seemed like dreams based on the reality taking place at my bedside. It was very important that friends and family continue to speak and elicit responses from me. I needed their interaction, even their foresight to play music or turn on the television. I look back and believe that I relied on their hope and their trust in prayer."[14] We have worked with many people in comas and know how difficult it can be to stay attuned with someone in coma. As helpers and family members we have a lot of duties and activities to perform, some of which are about attending to our patients' and loved ones' bodily needs. Structured by a tight time schedule, we have to perform many mechanical caregiving tasks. These are important and many families need more social and systemic support to perform them. But our roles as family members and caregivers go beyond the mechanical tasks. We need to believe in our love and relationship skills to overcome the communication barriers we face when our loved ones are unresponsive. Medicine has an ethical responsibility to support that aspect of care as well.

Can you imagine what it must be like to find yourself in a deep inner state with a glass wall that hinders your communication with the outside? In addition your sensory perceptions are altered, giving you unknown and possibly distorted information. You try to reach out but your body doesn't respond the way you intend it to. Your brain is injured and you don't have the same energy and "computing" reserves that you used to have. In such circumstances it is easy to understand that people's attentions and motivations would switch inward and that they might start to feel depressed and isolated, too.

Rehabilitation professionals working with people in comas understood the need for stimulation and have developed many stimulation practices. Multisensory stimulation is one such program that keeps coma patients stimulated with a series of audio, tactile, and visual impulses for hours each day. I have seen a program in Japan that bounced coma patients on trampolines, but to my knowledge there is no rehabilitation method that includes psychology and signal awareness to attune interventions to the patient's feedback and process. Process-oriented Coma Work integrates aspects of stimulation and reaching out to the deep inner and remote state of consciousness. Our subtle body work and communication skills allow us to find a way into the experiential world of a comatose person.

Imagine that you are a materialist and think and believe that consciousness or the mind is equivalent to and exclusively caused by brain activities. What do you think about a patient who has extensive damage to the brain? It seems obvious and reasonable that you would think that his or her mind won't work anymore as its most indispensable part, the brain machine, is broken. If the motor of your car is broken it's futile to think that you can drive the car. This materialist theory acts like a belief system and influences our thoughts, behaviors, and attitudes. It acts like voodoo or a curse on both patients and loved ones. As a 17-year-old boy was brought to the hospital in a deep coma, the neurosurgeon on duty remarked: "He won't live until morning and it's a good thing, because he'd be a vegetable." The young man recovered and recalled: "I remember him calling me a vegetable. I wouldn't move for him."[15] For this young man the hopeless attitude challenged him to rebel and paradoxically might have had a beneficiary result. But I know of many cases where such an attitude led to people retracting more deeply into the coma. Remember Erin from the Introduction? She had a history of depression and didn't have much support from her family. I still think that had a major role in her "poor" recovery. All our efforts had little effect. Even so, she briefly came out in one of my sessions.

You might retort that if the brain doesn't act like a machine, then many more patients should recover, so the fact that very few coma patients recover proves the mechanical theory. The question is what comes first? What is the impact of a mechanistic bias and resulting hopelessness? I, too, am sometimes skeptical and recognize the challenge of changing my own materialist views. It is very hard for us all to go beyond materialism or to add other views to our materialistic ones. What helped me is the direct experience I had with Erin. As I gradually learned to see brain and mind as two complementary expressions of a basic non-dual sentient reality, my perception, attitude, and behavior changed. The sentient realm is an experience that many mystics, shamans, and meditators have been exploring for centuries. Many of us seek that experience through mind-altering drugs. For others, these experiences may be frightening because they require us to go into altered states and we are afraid of losing the groundedness of consensus reality. One of our goals throughout this book is to help you to familiarize yourself with minimal altered states. These states act as preventive medicine and they will help you connect and relate to people in your environment who are in more serious altered states such as coma, vegetative, delusional or demented states.

Process-oriented Coma Work integrates recent knowledge from research on neuroplasticity. It addresses the consensus reality, that is, material and structural levels of coma (medical treatments, stimulation, and social issues) as well as the *process* and meaning of coma (through minimal communication signals, personal history, and family dynamics). Comatose people profit from state appropriate stimulation and from support for their teleological and goal-oriented process. Using stimulation techniques, joining the coma patient and communicating with him or her through tracking and unfolding their minimal cues, Process-oriented Coma Work enables us to tap into the comatose person's own healing motivation and enables optimal shaping and reorganization of new neural pathways and synaptic connections.

Placebo and the Biology of Hope

Above I have explained how beliefs and hopes play an important role in medicine and coma care. Now I will describe another process that demonstrates the significance of our psychology and beliefs for our health. Placebo describes the significant healing that results from the belief and expectation that you have received a powerful remedy, even if you were actually only given a sugar pill, saline water, or sham surgery. If you, your environment, and your caregivers believe in a certain treatment then the outcomes will be more positive than if you are convinced of the opposite, in which case you might experience more side effects or even harm from the treatment. Placebo effects clearly show that our brain activities can be influenced by our beliefs and expectations. Mental processes can be translated into neural brain events. From a purely materialist point of view, placebo effects do not make any sense. Materialism is unable to explain how this process whereby nonmaterial mental thoughts and feelings are translated into biophysical and chemical processes. However, it can be explained by a Process-oriented or *non-dualistic non-materialistic* model of medicine and illness that sees brain and mind as two complementary aspects of the same sentient reality: the *bodymind*, of which body and mind are each partial facets. Body and mind are complementary descriptions of a numinous sentient world. That fundamental imaginal realm manifests itself to us in both physical and mental ways; what we think and feel and what we experience in our bodies are expressions of the same sentient world. From a bodymind perspective, placebo means that encouragement, support, and hope are essential ingredients of any therapy. So psychology, the way you process issues, thoughts, and feelings is a crucial part of medicine and healing.

Dr. Bernard Lown,[16] a renowned cardiologist, provides many examples of the extraordinary powers of words—words that transcend the mechanical body, those that can injure and maim us, and words that can heal. One dazzling example is the case of a 60-year-old, critically ill man who recovered after he heard Dr. Lown referring to the galloping sound of his heart, which is paradoxically a bad prognostic sign in conditions of heart failure.

On Thursday morning, April twenty-fifth, you came in with your gang, surrounded the bed, and looked as though I was already in a casket. You put your stethoscope on my chest and urged everyone to listen to the "wholesome gallop." I figured that if my heart was still capable of a healthy gallop, I couldn't be dying, and I got well.[17]

In our current medical system, health professionals are trained to disclose all side effects and inform us about the possible dangers of any medical procedure and treatment. This is based on fears of litigation and legal issues. We are trained to provide realistic expectations and to discourage false hopes. For coma patients and their families for whom current thinking has little to offer, this has translated into a culture of hopelessness, isolation, and depression. From our Process-oriented point of view, this is another reason for the low recovery rates of people in persistent vegetative and minimally conscious states.

Medical Beliefs

Each person's and family's struggle with illness happens in a powerful field of beliefs. As we have seen, these beliefs can alter our experience and the outcome of our disease. Mainstream medicine in general regards the idea that illness can be a meaningful experience, as superfluous at best, and possibly even vaguely subversive. For the mainstream, psychology is perceived as a less important process that can influence behavior and treatment outcomes rather than as a fundamental component of all body functions and processes. Kleinman[18] describes an opposing view. He depicts mainstream medical views as an "iron cage" of medical beliefs that view the body simply as a machine. They are too technically narrow and therefore they dehumanize treatment. He sees engaging with the particular significances of a person's illness, and the stories in which patients reveal the meanings they attach to their suffering as a way for us to break out of the current limitations of medicine. Mindell's "Dreambody"[19] concept connects our subjective experience of bodily processes and diseases to symbols, roles, and patterns found in our night dreams, fantasies, and other altered state experiences. He opens the door to potentially enriching experiences and to the unfolding of extended meanings.

As I described earlier, meanings and explanations are by themselves significant and foster healing. Uncertainty, lack of control, and feeling one is at the mercy of random events are stressors that can lead to the breakdown of physiological functions. Giving a context, name, rationale, and significance to a process, which may otherwise feel frightening and out of our control, allows us to regain a measure of power and control. This is why many people feel relieved when they receive a diagnosis, even when that diagnosis is dreadful and the prognosis bad. Explanatory models and beliefs are a way out of the unknown into a meaningful and coherent context. Some of us may even go so far as to blame ourselves for a fateful disease, because it helps us to tolerate something that otherwise appears out of control or random. A diagnosis can be both a good and a bad thing. It can help us by giving us an explanation for a challenging process and it can also harm us.

A sense of coherence and minimal order is a physiological need. The explanations that people give to their body processes influence their behaviors in a powerful way. The explanations take all sorts of directions and can be both rational and very irrational. They are part of someone's "dreaming" and play an important part in the overall recovery process.

In addition, illness and suffering are also social experiences. Cultural values and collective modes of experience shape our individual perceptions and expressions. These culturally shaped patterns of how to relate to illness and disease are taught and learned via our socialization. Social and family interactions influence sick people's illness experience. For example, the grief and pain of family members for their loved one with supposedly terminal cancer may limit the person with the disease to the role of terminal cancer patient and thus co-create a negative outcome for the disease process. Negative expectations can be transmitted through health professionals' current health beliefs. They can have a great impact on patients' outcomes and chances for recovery. This nocebo effect is an ill effect caused by the *suggestion* or *belief* that something is harmful. In a landmark epidemiological study (the Framingham Heart Study), women who believed they were prone to heart disease were nearly four times as likely to die as women with similar risk factors who did not believe they were at risk.[20] Beliefs and expectations are strong medicine. Hope and hopelessness have direct effects on our bodies and our chances of recovery. Another example of this effect is when a new drug treatment is introduced with a huge marketing and advertising effort. They are promoted as the new solution for a certain disease and doctors and the public alike get very excited about the new hope for treating the disease. This cultural hype is part of the beneficial effect of the new treatment. Later, after a few years, when the treatment is not new and exciting anymore, the effectiveness of the drug diminishes.

The belief that someone's health will deteriorate or that someone will stay unconscious can be toxic. This is something that I continue to struggle with myself, to think that with my beliefs I participate in someone's health or disease process. What I think and what we think when we interact with someone in a certain process such as a comatose state shapes the course of that process. We are all entangled and synchronistically and non-locally connected[21] to each other. My point is that we need to understand the descriptive powers of belief systems; we need to develop our awareness about the impact of the ways we think about our bodies as individuals, families, and communities. Our beliefs help co-create medical outcomes both positive and negative. As helpers we need to notice which belief systems we and others are using, gain information about the forces in the field that our clients or patients are influenced by, and facilitate the awareness of and dialogue between these forces.

To summarize, it seems that our individual processes and experiences are influenced by the characteristic cultural meanings of time and place and the ways we consciously and subconsciously communicate them to each other. These cultural beliefs and moral values mingle with the sick person's subjective experience and shape his or her ability to heal and recreate a renewed sense of self and coherent view of his or her challenged life process.

Relevant Roles and Beliefs about Health

Every time and culture has specific beliefs about health. Everybody's illness experience is embedded in a social and cultural discourse about health. Today's beliefs and behaviors relating to the body and its suffering are linked to larger sociocultural dialogues. They are relevant for our individual disease processes because they inform our behaviors, what kind of treatment we choose, and what we do to stay healthy and prevent ourselves from getting sick. Our beliefs are also significant for us as family members, caregivers, and health professionals because they will communicate the hopes and expectations we have and influence the relationships between us. For example, if I think that illness might contain possible implicit positive meanings and growth potentials, I will react in a certain way to another care team or family member who sees the same process from a more mechanistic point of view.

While working with care teams and families taking care of someone in coma or with other serious health challenges, I often find that individuals will be polarized into taking certain roles and defending specific beliefs and values. As health professionals it is important to understand the various roles and polarities. They help us understand the family and relationship dynamics. Awareness of these roles can also help facilitate any tensions and conflicts that may arise. It is important to recognize that these roles are context specific. A specific family member might take a certain stance toward a care issue (for example, palliation or comfort care) when discussing the issue with medical providers and take another position when the same issue is talked about within the caregiver team or family. People will switch roles and viewpoints depending on the family or team constellation. The roles are important voices that need to be heard. It helps if we don't identify a specific role with a particular person.

Over time people's understanding of their health and bodies and their illness experience have circulated around polarized themes that often conflict with each other. The dialogue about health and medicine and the roles that represent the various sides are in all of us. All roles are needed, but once a role or belief dominates a specific situation, it will co-create the outcomes of an actual individual process. The more I study how people deal with health and disease processes the more I grow to believe that the various polarized roles reflect a deeper cultural struggle of getting to know ourselves and our bodies.

Examples of health-related themes that will polarize people are: nature or genes versus environment; individual responsibility versus collective or social causes; body versus mind; material versus spiritual; and objective disease versus subjective illness. I believe the debates about health are an ongoing group process that wants to awaken us to the many intertwined levels that influence our notions of health and disease. Together we are dreaming and unfreezing the essence of "health" and "illness" into life and being. The struggles between the many thoughts and beliefs about health and illness are, in my eyes, paradoxically an unwavering creative project that invites us to think more deeply about the issues at hand and to engage with spiritual and sentient aspects of life.

Asclepius, the Greek god identified with health and disease, and the first known physician, is often portrayed with a winged staff and two intertwined snakes that form a double-helix. This image has come to be the symbol of the modern physician, the caduceus (see Figure 3.1).

The caduceus is a helpful emblem for my contemplation of the evolution of the various roles. I conceive it as an ongoing dialogue between divergent polar conceptions, with singular themes: the snakes orbiting around a center of attraction and the rod symbolizing the stable and guiding sentient realm. I believe that the evolving dialogue between polar views of health brings to light new facets of universal human problems, and thus allows us to deepen our understanding of these essential issues, and of ourselves. Coma, coma recovery stories, end-of-life care issues, assisted suicide, and the withdrawal of life-sustaining treatment measures are themes that receive a lot of press. As a culture we are learning to understand the complexities of these existential problems.

Let me now explore in more detail some specific health-related polarized themes.

Material versus Nonmaterial/Spiritual

One culturally prevalent belief system that we all carry is the separation between the everyday world of practical activities and the spiritual world. From this perspective disease can be symbolic of the relationship

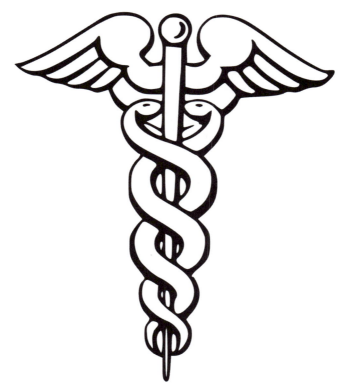

Figure 3.1 The Caduceus
(Courtesy of Wikimedia at http://en.wikipedia.org/wiki/File:Caduceus.svg)

between the spiritual and the practical. When we get sick or depressed we are forced out of our ordinary everyday reality. We can't function and pursue our practical activities. We are forced to slow down, rest, become altered, and possibly reconnect with other dimensions in our lives that our practical selves have marginalized. If we open ourselves up to this alternative world we can find hidden treasures of renewed creativity and meaning.

From a spiritual perspective a possible explanation of illness is non-natural causes (such as fate or destiny) and being sick is seen in moral terms (the individual is imperfect and challenged to learn). "Spiritual" paradigms can assume an individual or collective form. Illness may be linked to the fundamentally faulty nature of man, and humans are exhorted to strive to better themselves. Alternatively, illness may be believed to be caused by individually and collectively broken "taboos" or restrictions. Unhealthy habits or behaviors such as excessive smoking and drinking or not being concerned about diet are overlaid with cultural moral judgments, and many people will feel guilty and have a bad conscience when engaging in such behaviors. Disease is a corruption that indicates our imperfections and limitations, but also it creates occasional insight and knowledge.

The material role, on the other hand, lives in the world of natural causes, mediated by physical agents such as viruses or social and environmental factors, and the individual is not held accountable. This is the realm of materialist Cartesian beliefs that define illness as a malfunction of the human machine. The material view, however, predates Descartes, as even the early Greeks believed that health and illness had mechanical explanations. For them various outer or inner forces disrupted the balance of basic elements and structures. Illness was a consequence of an excess of one element and a lack of balance. This notion of balance then leads to a set of ethical values in which a good life is expressed through moderation and avoidance of excess. Most modern prescriptions of exercise and diet are based on this mechanical concept of a balanced life style.

Here is an exercise (Exercise 3.1) to help you explore your own health related beliefs.

Rational versus Emotional

We have all internalized this polarity to some degree, and in our minds and actions we often separate between rationality or reason and emotions. The emotional and impulsive nature of human beings stands in contrast to rational and reasonable thoughts and behaviors. One side holds the value of cognitive thinking, making rational decisions, and being practical and reasonable. The other side favors feelings, intuitions, dreaming, and creativity. These values and attitudes are often polarized along stereotypical

Exercise 3.1
Health Beliefs

1. Recall the last time you had the flu. Remember the state the flu forced you into. Describe it in a few words. Find the energy of that flu state. Express it with a hand motion or an energy sketch on a piece of paper.
2. Find the role, identity, or part of yourself that this energy is against or that suffers from it. Describe this energy of your usual/normal self. Express it with a hand motion or an energy sketch.
3. What are the beliefs and values of both roles or experiences? How do they differ from each other? With a friend or in your mind, role play both sides of the discussion. Which side are you, usually, and why? What is against one or the other side?

gender lines, women being more identified with the soft skills of emotions and men representing the hard skills of practicality and so-called realism. This polarity also extends to projections onto whole professions: medicine often being identified with objectifiable processes, whereas psychology embarks on the quest to understand the subjective, subtle, and elusive intrapersonal and interpersonal relationships. In coma care teams and families, these two roles often surface and conflict with each other—for example, in decisions about end-of-life care, continuation of care, choosing treatment options, etc.; these roles will represent opposing sides. Often they will be represented by people in specific gender and/or professional roles. In coma care, female nurses will often argue for the value of more quality care, touch, massage, music, and talking to the person while male doctors will more often stress the value of more invasive treatments, diagnostic explorations, or the withdrawal of treatment.

Kleinman, Das, and Lock[22] claim that Christian monotheism has had a determinative influence on Western biomedicine. The idea of a single God and the imperative of a universal moral order led to the dominance of rational principles and the idea of a single objective truth. It also fostered a single-minded approach to illness and care with an extreme insistence on materialism as the foundation of knowledge and a consistent marginalization of the role of subjectivity and feelings. Mainstream medicine, developed on the base of Cartesian materialism, has a very strong value orientation, sees nature as purely physical, and is devoid of any teleological meaning. That serious illness may involve a quest for meaning is disavowed. The positive aspect of this reductionist approach has been the development of biochemical-oriented technology and its many successes in the treatment of acute pathology. But by proceeding within this cultural logic of dualistic opposition between male and female, mind and body, hard and soft, strength and weakness, technology and human experience, biomedicine has sanctioned the ongoing marginalization of the "softer" side of the poles. Following that logic, "soft" medical procedures and specialties, which concentrate on the human practice of medicine and seek to understand its social, psychological, and moral aspects have low value, provide the lowest incomes, and attract more women practitioners. And many coma patients who are seen as beyond the reach of hard skills and rely mainly on softer skills are also marginalized and neglected. Many end up in nursing facilities without adequate specialized care.

The rational worldview, which is deemed necessary for a scientific conception and analysis of nature, nevertheless, has not yet permeated all aspects of life and society. Spiritual, shamanistic, or mystical beliefs are still very prevalent in many tribal cultures around the world. They also remain very influential in our perceptions of ailments that lack obvious scientific or causal explanations. Confronted with disturbing symptoms that doctors can't explain, many people will relate their symptoms to repressed thoughts and preoccupations. Magical or archetypal thinking, irrational fears, and the association of emotions and feelings with disease and their cures are features of this "spiritual" thinking. In my view both approaches are valuable and both have been hurtful and helpful over time. More recent debates in medical practice are striving for integrating the pre-existing polarities of the material and spiritual views of the body and medicine, as well as the mechanical and more sentient aspects of disease and illness.

In recent years many scientific studies have been conducted on distance healing and the effects of prayer or meditation on medical treatment. The numinous realm has become part of a scientific endeavor. Increasingly research is being done on the biology of religious/spiritual experience in an attempt to learn how physiology connects with spiritual experiences.[23] In the West the issue of religion and science has long been perceived as an either/or dichotomy, which presumes that the two poles exist only in opposition to each other. In academic medicine, spirituality and science have largely been seen as two opposing paradigms with the exception of the new developments mentioned above. However, for other cultures and in the lived experience of many people, they were never that separate. The empirical and spiritual components of medicine have always evolved in intertwined strands. In its immediacy, illness is always experienced as a disorder of both the material and biological body, and as a disruption of the sentient, or spiritual, body.

THE BODY'S SENTIENT ASPECTS

The first characteristic of the living body is that of sentience. The very meaning of our bodies is that they are animated by subjective feelings and sensations. These subtle sensations of pressure and tension give us a sense of where one's body is in space, as well as an immediate sense of connectedness to the body. These sensorimotor experiences also distinguish the lived body from all other physical objects. They provide us with a primary "knowing," that is, a "knowing" through the body. This subtle "knowing" from within is what connects us to the sentient world ("the Tao that cannot be spoken") as basic reality.

One aspect of every disease process is that it interrupts our sense of integrity, the taking for granted of the body. Illness draws attention to the material nature of the body and is experienced as a disruption of the sentient body—a disruption that includes an altered experience of space and time, changes in self-image and self-identity, and threats to social roles and status.

With his Dreambody concept, Arnold Mindell[24] founded the new school of Process-oriented Psychology. He discovered that dreams and body experiences come together, that every nighttime dream is connected to a body experience and that every body experience can be visualized and usually appears in a dream.[25] If a symptom feels like a pressure it is likely that people or characters who pressure you will appear in your dreams. Later Arnold Mindell expanded his Dreambody concept by incorporating quantum physics into his research about body symptoms and medicine.[26] He was interested in the question of how a symptom, such as pressure, felt *before* it became such an intense symptom. He found out that the subtle feeling experiences at the core of a symptom experience related to the deeper psychological and spiritual aspects of a person's identity and process. At that essence or *process wisdom*[27] level, the spiritual and the material come together. He differentiates between the everyday world of practical activities in which consensual views of reality reign and a more symbolic numinous realm that is governed by more dreamlike events. Symptoms are seen as an attempt to compensate for the one-sidedness of consensual reality and as a link to the world of sentient experiences. Mainstream views structure our experience of normality, what we perceive as functional or dysfunctional, normal or deviant, healthy or unhealthy. They influence the way we feel about certain groups of people (for example, coma patients or the elderly) and various types of bodies (for example, the thin and the obese body, the healthy or diseased body). The doctrines that arise from the social dialogue are subjected to power struggles within competing social groups and interests with some dominating over others and defining what counts as "truth."

From a Process Work standpoint the most marginalized aspect of today's discourse about life and our experience of it is the realm of bodymind or sentience. Materialistic views dominate our current perception and experience of reality. From quantum physics Mindell extrapolates a dimension of experience in which time is nonlinear and parts, events, and ideas are entangled and non-local. In this sentient dimension basic tendencies, moods, and atmospheric changes reign. Subtle influences and energies resonate throughout our bodies and manifest in slight discomforts and symptoms at the fringe of our awareness. They can later develop into full-blown symptoms and diseases.

Asclepius's rod is a good metaphor for this sentient realm. The rod stands for the core from which the dreaming manifests. From a central core the manifold themes unfold as polarities and dichotomies and in creating tension and diversity they bring forth consciousness and awareness. The two intertwined snakes awaken us to the complexities of health. They stand for dualistic thinking whose strength is to raise the polarities and help us explore these issues. The rod represents the complementary aspect of seemingly opposing approaches, the sentient realm of interconnectedness in which there are no rigid boundaries between things, thoughts, people, and events. In the cultural debate the rod as the unifying sentient experience has been marginalized.

Polar mechanistic and spiritual concepts are opposite sides of the same coin. Both views emerge from a deeper level, the fecund field of sentience from which everything arises. The rod is the root foundation out of which matter and the power that gives rise to the matter emerge. From a sentient perspective there is no such thing as inert material. Every object, cell, and body is full of scintillating potentialities. From this viewpoint even the most materialistic aspects of disease processes— like test results documenting physiological or biochemical processes— have dreamlike qualities that mirror their sentient origin.

Process-oriented views of illness and coma are holistic and the methods we use to facilitate the learning and growth opportunity integrate mechanistic and sentient approaches. The patients' and families' subjective experience is what guides us in our interventions. Symptoms have very subjective qualities; pain, for example, can be experienced as throbbing, dull, sharp, or burning and can change over time. My own asthma symptoms have changed in their qualities. I used to have more allergic reactions but just now they are mostly exercise-induced. They force me to slow down and move very intently. If I change my pace and engage in walking meditation they disappear. My current life situation is characterized by pressure, pressure to finish this book and pressure to organize a big international conference. But if I follow my asthma's guidance, and slow down and meditate, I am reminded of my transient nature and my own expectations become less dominant. In my visualization I see myself as one pawn in a larger attempt to change a medical paradigm. My symptoms take me out of my ordinary self and momentary situation.

The example of my asthma symptoms reveals another aspect of our work with body symptoms. Every body symptom is characterized by two different partial experiences. The direct subjective experience of the symptom, such as the tightness and pressure I feel from my asthma, and the "emotional" state I experience as a reaction to or consequence of my symptom, which in my example is the meditative state that I go into if I follow my symptom. Examples of clients' subjective accounts are: "There is a drilling inside my head," "a red hot poker feeling that is constant and in my head, my jaw," "a pressure that wants to come out of my body," etc. Examples of clients' descriptions of their emotional states are: "I feel empty and scared of the future," "I cry a lot and don't care anymore," "I am very angry at doctors," "I am very nervous and stressed." Emotional states include anger, shame, and guilt, and can be symptoms of depression and anxiety. The emotional states also describe relationship processes between the clients and their environment: their experience of feeling marginalized or misunderstood by family members or members of the care team and community. The emotional states can also be triggered by internalized conflicts with an inner critic or an expression of internalized outer expectations. All these are aspects of psychological work with people who suffer from body symptoms.

Exercise 3.2 will help you have an experience of what I am describing. Use your own creativity and intuition in following the steps. There is no right or wrong way. The whole goal is to gain more understanding and awareness.

One of our biggest problems is that we think we ought to be this or that. In so doing we marginalize other aspects of ourselves, and symptoms become something we don't agree with. Besides addressing the consensus reality difficulties that symptoms have and using medicine, exercise, massage, herbal supplements, etc., you can also use the exercise below to help you befriend another aspect of your symptom and to show you that the dreaming process in your symptom is meaningful.

Exercise 3.2
Unfolding a Body Symptom

1. Think about one of your own symptoms right now, or a symptom that you had in the past that you would like to understand better.
2. Where is or was the symptom? What does or did that symptom feel like?
3. If you remember a recent dream, which person or character personifies the energy or quality of the symptom?
4. Express the symptom energy with a gesture or hand motion.
5. Explore the emotional state or mood that the symptom creates in you.
6. Follow the symptom energy back to its origin or essence. Find the subtle feeling that is at the core of the more intense symptom. One way to get to that essence is by imagining acting out the symptom energy (e.g., the pressure) and then slowly doing it less and less to get to the initial intent of the energy.
7. Try to embody that initial intent. What does it say to you?
8. How are the symptom energy, the emotional state, and the essence energy inter-related?

The Process-oriented approach to symptoms is nonpathological; rather it is curious about the potential learning that you can gain from any experience, including body symptoms and comatose states.

Comatose people are in an extremely different place. For them and their families everything is disrupted. The only remaining link to the outside world is through their sentient bodies and their subtle signals and reactions. There aren't any simple exercises that we can guide them through or any firm rules for working with them. Everything is a process; it depends on the moment, the state of the comatose person and the signals that come from him or her, the belief systems of the families and care teams, and the feedback you receive from the comatose person and the caregivers. Again, on a consensus reality level, there is trauma, someone not responding in conventional ways, many medical and caregiving questions, many financial and social issues, and so forth. On another level, there is someone who is going through a process and having experiences that need our support and facilitation. And there is also a family that is part of that process and in need of guidance.

Both Terry Wallis and Rom Houben[28] were both thought to be brain dead for 20 years. But then, Terry suddenly addressed his mother as "Mom!" and Rom's doctors discovered that he was very much awake. Current research says that up to 40 percent of those thought to be in a persistent vegetative state are, in fact, quite conscious.[29] All of these people are conscious but no one realizes it. They have to listen to people say that they are as good as dead. Their families give up and drop them, too, because everybody says there is no one home. Process-oriented Coma Work offers the sensitive tools to bridge the gap between people in nonresponsive states and the outside world.

WHAT IS HEALING?

Gary: Pierre does a wonderful job of talking about different scientific ways of approaching this whole area of healing and health and the way science and Process Work interface. I would like to add to the discussion by bringing in some of what I have learned from my clients.

Jeff is in a hospital on the East Coast. A young man in his thirties, he suffered from an aneurysm in the middle of the night. He was without oxygen to his brain for an undetermined, but significant amount of time. When I saw him, he was medically stabilized, but his family had been told that he had no chance of any kind of recovery. They were told specifically that those parts of his brain related to cognition, speech, and movement had been destroyed, and, of course, all of the medical tests that had been done backed up this prognosis. His wife and mother were hopeless. Jeff stayed in his bed in the hospital most of the time, except when he was put in a wheelchair, when the family could wheel him around. We were called in after he had been in the coma for about six months. I began by assessing him and saw that his responses to all of my interventions were very minimal. After about two hours' worth of work, the most feedback I saw was that his right eye had opened briefly. I asked the family if there was anything that they had done that produced more of a response. The mother said that sometimes, up in the chair, Jeff would keep both eyes open for a minute or two. We worked with him all morning, to little avail, and then went to lunch. When we came back, Jeff was in his chair, and his family said we could take him out to the lobby. The nurses came by several times, and in spite of the fact that I had medical clearance to work with Jeff, they made comments to the family about how they were wasting their time and money, and even told the family I was a fake. The family looked even more skeptical. I was stuck—the feedback had been extremely minimal. I tried to drop into my deepest self and into my body to find something that was guiding me beyond all the external pressures. Suddenly, I had an idea. I was helping Jeff to gently stretch one arm that was all locked up. He was in a wheelchair, and I had this idea to stretch him by gently moving the chair in circles, so I moved him around me with his arms gently stretched, as if were dancing together. I had recently seen a massage practitioner do a beautiful circular massage in a swimming pool with someone, and I wondered what would happen if I kept making circles. As I begin to gently turn him, Jeff's eyes open wider and wider. He kept them open, as long as I kept moving him. When I stopped, his eyes closed. When a colleague did some very helpful bodywork on him, that is work that would have been helpful if he were in a waking state or if it were his process to have that kind of body work, he didn't open his eyes again for two hours. Later I began to turn him and move him again, and his eyes stayed open not just for two minutes, but for most of a two-hour period.

Jeff, like most coma patients, was generally kept quiet and not stimulated very much. When I ask families why they do so little with their loved ones, their response is that they have been told that the person needs rest and quiet. I understand the need for rest, especially immediately after an accident when the body does most of its physical healing. However, if I am still being told this when the person has been in coma for six months, I think it is time to try something else. So I just kept turning Jeff and moving him. I made lots of excited and playful sounds while I did this, and he kept looking very interested in what was happening. I stretched his arm gently and used this stretch to move him around my body in his chair. When he seemed bored, I would modify what I was doing. That night Jeff and I were both tired, so I went home to have some dinner and sleep, but as soon as I arrived home, I received a call from Jeff's wife Laura saying that something utterly astounding had happened. They were about to put Jeff back in bed and Laura asked him if he was ready. She had regularly asked him questions like this in the past, and had never had a response. Suddenly Jeff said "Yes, I am tired." Laura ran and got the nurse, who heard Jeff again say "Yes" and also respond "No" to another question. Laura called me in half excitement, half panic. Jeff had started talking, which had thrilled her, but he had stopped talking again right after that, which sent her into a panic that he might never speak again! We worked with him for a few more days, and he said a few more words. Over the next few weeks, he was able to move a ball with his arms, and showed other signs of progress. Currently, I am supervising other therapists working with Jeff, and they are working on some of the psychological issues present before his coma, which seemed to be playing themselves out in his recovery. The family is still very frustrated that he hasn't healed more, but considering his prognosis, I keep telling the therapists to reassure them that this is certainly significant progress, and that healing like this can take years.

There is one final note that adds to the flavor of this particular piece of Coma Work. The day after Jeff began to speak, several of the nurses gathered around me, the same ones who had told his wife I was a fraud, because there was nothing that could be done for him. This time they told me that I was a very good doctor, and then walked out of the room. Something else had changed; not only had Jeff changed, but the atmosphere at the hospital had changed, too.

These are the main lessons I learned, or had reinforced, from working with Jeff. Although I came from a practical rather than a theoretical angle, I came to many of the same conclusions as Pierre did earlier in this chapter.

1. Once a medical diagnosis is made, this leads to a prognosis of chances of recovery. However, a prognosis, especially when it involves the brain, is only a prediction about what some, or most people will do. Prognoses around brain damage recovery do not currently include what might happen when Process-oriented body-mind interventions are introduced.

2. Diagnoses and prognoses tend to be self-fulfilling prophecies. If families and medical staff see someone as having no potential for recovery, this will influence how they treat the person both directly and indirectly. Even if

something new happens, like when I showed up with a different method, the prognosis makes the person trying different interventions look like a fraud. Many of the families I have worked with, who haven't given up on their loved ones, have been told by medical staff that they need to get over their denial and move on. Sometimes this is great advice and is just the support that the family needs to let go, but at other times, it is really the professional saying "I am at the limit of what I can do, so therefore I think there is no hope for your loved one." If it were said this way, then the family could see this as the practitioner's limits rather than nature's limits, and so they may feel freer to explore alternatives.

3. The "right method" for the client may be a prescribed method, such as allopathic medicine, acupuncture, chiropractic or naturopathic methods, or may be something mysterious that emerges out of the particular client's process. In Jeff's case, the answer to the question, "What is healing?" would be spinning him for hours, and then moving him back and forth from one end of the room to another in a wheelchair. It defied all the methods the allopathic and naturopathic people were treating him with. In fact, what I did was even way over my ordinary mind's limits. Something came through me that allowed me to do something safe and radical, spinning him like this, slowly turning together for hours, like we were in some kind of sacred Dervish ritual. Why did moving Jeff in circles work? Mostly it's a mystery, there are so many possibilities and I can only speculate. Perhaps he needed movement work because he was stuck inside himself in feeling states, and the movement helped him to come out. Methods that helped him feel his body more, such as hands-on work, put him deeper into the state. When Jeff first started going into the state that culminated in his aneurysm, he began to thrash around. So movement was part of his symptom, and maybe the circular movements helped to complete something that was beginning when the symptom happened. In Process Work theory, we say that symptoms happen at the edge of personal development, whether in seeing, hearing, feeling, moving, relating, being connected to the world or to spirit. Perhaps he had reached to a movement edge, and the spinning got him moving again. Why circular movement? Circular movement has always been associated with play in children, and with altered states in adults. Groups like the whirling dervishes, a Sufi spiritual order, spin themselves around and around until they go into ecstasy. Perhaps spinning gave him access to altered states that helped him come out of coma, or that replaced the need for the more permanent altered state of the coma. What we can say, that is measurable here, is that there was a change in Jeff. He was completely nonresponsive and that day he talked. We can also explain how to do these kinds of interventions. I know from talking to many close friends and family members who are traditional physicians that all kinds of intuitive experiences come through them. We can all be trained to trust the value of both our formal rational training and the beauty and wisdom of our intuitive knowledge.

4. Don't give up if the institution, the doctors, nurses, and rest of the staff act questioningly, or put down the work you are doing with the person in coma. Paradigm shifts don't come easily. People generally perceive reality based on the way they have been trained, and in which they are highly invested in maintaining as a valid practice. And yet, in the background for many in the field of Coma Work, there is a longing for something that works better than the present tools and methods. So whenever I have been able to be patient and relate to the concerns of the institutions, there has always been at least one person on the staff, perhaps a doctor, nurse, physiotherapist, or speech therapist, who gets interested and becomes supportive of what I am doing. Be aware of success though. I often expected to be appreciated and embraced if people came out of the coma. However the few times I have been asked to leave a hospital by a physician were when the patient had been making good progress or had made a major breakthrough. Once when a physician higher up in the hierarchy than the one the family had received permission from had heard the buzz about our work and what was happening, we were asked to leave immediately. This might have been prevented by being more careful to ensure that the family had asked for permission as high up in the command chain as necessary to work there. However, we might still have been thrown out despite perfect permission, because to embrace what we are saying would require a major shift in thinking, and it raises difficult issues about the kind and quality of care generally offered in the hospital. I understand this position completely. Imagine how you would feel if you were running one of the top coma hospitals in the world. Suddenly someone comes and works in the way I work, and questions are raised about whether or not it is OK to leave patients alone without any stimulation or interaction or deep processing. This would be a shock to your identity, as maybe you are not running a hospital that is as fantastic as you thought it was, and you may actually have to look at whether you are missing the boat. It might be easier not to look at this, at least as for as long as it is possible to avoid facing such a different reality.

In a way, institutions are also in comas. They are asleep to what might be missing in their care and work with people, and I need to be a coma worker with them, too, and follow their process about how to awaken them to this new direction. Some may say never. Others may say as soon as I see more research, and still others will say slowly, slowly, through building relationships and over time I will take a bit of what you have to offer.

On the other hand, I know things are definitely changing. In 2004, Pierre and I were invited to present our Process-oriented Coma Work to the alternative medical community connected with Dr. Andrew Weil at the University of Arizona Medical School. And I have recently been approached by a group of scientists from Israel interested in studying what we do and why it works. I have also had several doctors approach me about working with their loved ones, and that certainly indicates an openness to look beyond the allopathic box.

I am also interested in institutions and organizational development, so if I am asked to leave I try to go back and process the conflict with the administrative people who have asked me to leave, including physicians if they are willing. One told me not to bother trying to change things because he was retiring and therefore wanted to leave things be. Another told me he needed more research that validated what we were doing. Still another told me he was very open and interested in my methods, and needed me to do more to ensure that his hospital was covered around liability. I had all the necessary insurance coverage; he just needed more documentation to feel safe. I want to recommend to families and to professionals to enter into dialogues with the physicians if they initially say no to this kind of Coma Work, because through dialogue I have always found more openness than was initially apparent.

Jeff's case raises many questions that need further exploration, but I want to highlight one of the most important issues raised here. Why does someone come part way back, but not all the way? Why in this case, if Jeff can talk, does he rarely do so? Why does he make so much progress in thinking, but less in speaking, and even less in movement? If according to standard medical understanding he shouldn't be able to make progress in any area, why does he make the patterns of progress he makes? Is it something in him, or is it what we do as his caregivers? Are we missing some major signals in his process, or is he teaching us that some progress is enough progress, or that getting back to normal is not so important?

Another central issue this case raises is what does relationship have to do with all of this? Jeff had his aneurysm in the middle of a relationship battle. Another man I worked with had his heart attack the day after a major relationship hurt. It is easy for me to understand how something very hurtful or shocking can put the body into so many traumas that it shuts down. What is more difficult to understand, though, is how does healing these issues while in the coma help? For instance, in one case one person told a loved one, shortly before his stroke, that she really didn't love him, and then afterward told him over and over again how she had learned that she really did love him, but he didn't respond. Why not when another person in a similar situation did respond? Maybe coma resembles ordinary waking consciousness in that sometimes someone apologizes and it helps everything to return to a positive state, and sometimes sorry is just too late and the damage is done. Much more research needs to be done on this and on the whole issue of coma and depression. The vast majority of people I have worked with in coma had been in a significant depression within the year before their coma, and this is obviously a much higher rate than in the general population. Perhaps relationship difficulties are a subset of the whole area of depression and coma that needs to be looked into.

My own approach values all of the knowledge that alternative healing has for us, as well as the more intuitive, nonrational realms. I value the technical healer in all of us and the shaman, and I would like to see these parts come closer together and cooperate more, for our own and our client's benefit. Coma is not just about returning the person to their previous life, but is an attempt to make a leap in consciousness. Sometimes the person can bring their experiences back and integrate them into their ordinary life, their family, and culture. But sometimes this leap in consciousness, I believe, frees the person to die and to finish up their work in this life. And at other times this leap becomes a long-term state that cooks the person slowly and thoroughly. It is our job as process workers to facilitate the coma process so as to make things as fluid and easy as possible for the person and their loved ones.

Pierre: There are also many medical traditions around the world that are less dualistic and more open to competing paradigms and that seem less troubled by the uncertainty of human experience. For example, Taoists understood the cyclic nature of the world. In their thinking, the dynamic contrasts and polarities don't form independent units but are, like Yin and Yang, components of the bodymind. They are in complementary relationship and in a continuous flow.

The symbol of the ouroboros (the snake biting its own tail) and the metaphor of the dancing Shiva, who with one hand creates the world only to destroy it with the other, both also describe this melting pot of complementary opposites, which balance each other rather than being in opposition to each other. "They arise together, depend on each other while they exist, and perish together."[30] Body processes are additionally regarded as being in close interaction with the Yin and Yang constituents of the collective and of nature. In India, for example, the body-mind is held to be permeable to substances and symbols in social interactions. Health in this context is viewed as a balance between the body and the constituents of the outer world. And, as I mentioned earlier, in parts of ancient Western society a similarly dialectical or balanced view existed of body, self, and world. Furthermore, many of these cultures also perceive bodily complaints as collective moral problems: they are symbols of disharmonies in social relationships and in culture.

Each medical tradition has its own validity and no one tradition covers all the different aspects of human suffering. It seems clear that Western health sciences offer powerful tools for understanding and treating many different conditions and open up new possibilities for positive change. On the other hand, its dominant scientific and medical language reinforces dualistic worldviews and devalues patients' sense of wholeness. Biomedical materialism has no place for God or the soul and views matter as being totally inert. It disproved the concept of vitalism, and refutes the existence of a vital power or life force. This thinking has proved enormously successful for certain purposes in certain areas. But in this disenchanted worldview there is no place for mystery or magic; with the demise of the divine and the numinous realm and with the denial of our sentient experiences and our dreaming nature, all of our inner experiences, which follow alternative values to those of objective materialism, are marginalized. If we deny the idea of a life force that animates our bodies and selves, there is no way to tap into the therapeutic powers within ourselves, which, when we connect to them, can help us regain strength and overcome fatigue and sickness.

Based on his Dreambody concept and his understanding of quantum mechanics, Arnold Mindell[31] proposes a new holistic approach to medicine and body experiences. He developed many tools and skills for unraveling the subjective meanings underneath our bodily complaints that I am not going to describe in detail here. To conclude, I would like to focus on the question of how an integrated view of health translates into our own everyday lived experience. Most of us will, while we are healthy, direct our attention outward toward our involvements in the world and our bodies will remain largely unnoticed and taken for granted. Our bodies stay in the background of our awareness. Our conscious focus is toward meeting the challenges of everyday life, and we marginalize the subtle dreaming aspects of our living bodies and their primarily sentient characteristics. In sickness, when our symptoms submerge us, our bodies suddenly become the foreground. When faced with symptoms, most of us will probably initially display a medical reflex in which we seek restitution and cure. This is the first step. Nobody will be open to go deeper into understanding and learning from their experience if they can't get relief first. But from our experience, illness is not only an enemy that needs to be defeated but also an opportunity for increased awareness and growth. The things that we are against and the irritations we experience in illness also have a nonpathological side to them that are meaningful. We suggest doing both fighting *and* opening ourselves up to learning. It takes courage and discipline to learn from something that we are basically against. It is not always possible. But it is worth trying.

I suggest a medical culture in which we relearn an empathic understanding of our bodies and an experiential awareness of the sentient

Exercise 3.3
Exploring Our Subtle Body Tendency

1. Put your book aside, sit back, and relax. Take a moment to notice your body and how it feels right now to be in it. Notice your breathing and other subtle feelings. Don't try to change anything, just notice.
2. Next notice the subtle tendency that your body has to move in a certain direction. Notice where it wants to go. Is it leaning to one side or another? Wanting to go up or down?
3. Begin to follow this natural tendency to move. Allow it to guide you. Be moved by your body's inherent intelligence. Follow the movement until somehow the process feels completed.
4. Put words to your experience. What is your body telling you? How is your experience at the end of the exercise different from the beginning?

feelings that animate our bodies. One way to enhance experiential consciousness of the body's "dreaming" is by engaging in embodied practices such as sentient proprioceptive inner work. Sentient meditation on the body brings the lived body into our conscious awareness. In this practice we are directed to turn our attention to the immediate experience of our bodies and to discover the subtle feelings that permeate them. This sentient symptom work is a way to tune into the dreamsong of our bodies and to explore the essential life force that gives our lives meaning and direction. Empathic listening requires that we give our bodies' stories ongoing attention rather than only when symptoms overflow our awareness.

Here is an exercise (Exercise 3.3) to give you an experience of this sentient proprioceptive inner work.

Everybody's lived experience is complex and multifaceted. It isn't limited to an either/or approach nor to the rational and objective truth stance of Western medicine and science. In our lived experience many different perspectives can all be true at the same time and interconnectedness is a basic reality. From this perspective every disease is both spiritual and material. The distinctions are helpful because they nourish the group processing that is necessary for increased consciousness and awareness. But ultimately all factors need to be accepted and included as part of any disease process; the sentient realm of the rod as well as the intertwined snakes that symbolize the manifold polarities. Our lived reality has both a material foundation and a nonvisible and nonvisualizable dimension of pure generative power. Symptoms in their material and subjective expression are, from this perspective, not only a source of suffering and pain, but also an unseen ocean of creative potentialities.

Chapter 4

The Mystery of Relationship in Coma Care and Recovery

This chapter covers the various relationship issues that might be affected by having a loved one in coma and how relationship issues within caregiver teams might affect the person in coma. We discuss relevant relationship issues that might precede coma and when someone awakens from coma. We also include information about working with the family and relationship issues in the moment at the coma person's bedside and include exercises that explore these issues and help loved ones and caregivers work on them.

WHAT DO RELATIONSHIPS AND COMA HAVE TO DO WITH EACH OTHER?

Gary: People in comas are like the rest of us around relationship. All possible combinations of interest and disinterest can be present in the person in coma. Some seem interested in relationship before coma, but not during. Others are interested both before and during coma. Still others weren't interested in relationship before coma, and became interested during coma, and finally some seem totally disinterested in relationship all the time. The coma state makes it very clear what people are and aren't interested in, so it exaggerates the normal sense of presence or nonpresence in a relationship. In this chapter, we will look at relationships and coma in general and also at how to work with relationships in coma.

I want to begin by bringing in here the writing I have previously done on family therapy with the coma patient, *Vital Loving* (2004). I have revised this work to include new developments in Process Work and Process-oriented Coma Work. I will then add specific details around one-on-one relationship work and relationship work in general when in coma.

Coma is one of the most intense physical symptoms a family can experience. Working with the family of someone in a coma brings us literally to the edge between life and death. Working so close to this edge requires special approaches, which can help us learn new ways to work with other family situations where a member faces physical death. Loving someone at the gate of life and death is part of what vital loving is all about.

One of the most painful experiences I hear from family members and people who come out of a coma is that they couldn't find anyone with whom to address the psychological and spiritual issues a coma brings with it. Process-oriented Coma Work is based on the central belief that a coma is a meaningful part of the individual's development. The person is seen as having important and often profound experiences in this state. By using special bodymind techniques, a therapist can connect with the person in a coma and help them make use of the state. This work may also help people recover more quickly, and in some cases, they may come out of the coma.

I have spent hundreds of hours sitting with the families of people in a coma, often at the bedside of the coma patient. Sometimes I work with the family huddled in the waiting room at an intensive care unit, or, in the later stages of a coma, at someone's home or at a nursing home. Several important themes emerge from this type of work.

COMA AS AN AMPLIFIER OF EXISTING FAMILY PATTERNS

The first principle of family work with one family member in a coma is that this extreme situation tends to amplify previous feelings toward the person in a coma and can therefore bring more awareness to family patterns of relating and provide an opportunity to process these issues and experiences. In one family I worked with, where the young man in a coma, Sandy, was clearly loved, family members sat with him every moment the hospital would allow. Six months into his coma, his bed was still surrounded not only by parents and siblings, but also by grandparents, aunts, and cousins. This family consulted with me and with other experts in Coma Work and developed their own kind of coma therapy that produced good results. When an emergency department physician saw Sandy six months after his accident, he was stunned by the progress being made in such a severe head injury-related coma. The family had been told that Sandy probably would never come out of the coma. However, when he ended up in the emergency department for another medical problem, he actually did come out of the coma. He was disoriented at first and subsequently needed a great deal of rehabilitation, but at that moment in the emergency department, he was suddenly speaking and then screaming. Up until that point he had slowly been making progress, and then some combination of the therapy, plus the withdrawal of certain medications due to the medical crisis, allowed him to come out of the coma. The family believed in him and in the medical system and kept going with him.

Once out of the coma, there was still much work to do. One of the concerns about him in coma was his blood pressure spikes and the medicine he was taking to regulate it. However, when he came out, he would often pound his fist into the wall. I wonder how much his blood pressure was connected to his pent-up anger and the pounding on the wall. One way or another way this family had to work with this part of their son and therefore this part of themselves. The father was a very interesting man in that he was a former military person who now fought for peace as a peace activist. On several occasions the mother became very angry with me. The whole family was dancing with this energy of anger that needed to find a way to work itself out. Watching this young man was like watching a theater of anger. He had such a violent auto accident and was thrown hundreds of feet from the car. Now, looking back, with the advancements we have made in this work, I would have showed him these two sides of himself and the family. There is the angry one and the peaceful one, the blood pressure and the blood pressure medicine. The sides were dancing together. Apparently the medicine was doing something to his liver that produced a crisis. If I had known then, as I do now, how to have this dialogue with and for him, his liver may not have had to have the discussion. I would have dropped down into my center and put the violent side and the peaceful side each in one hand, and then worked to put the two together. I would have let the two sides work themselves out through me. Then I would have found a way to put the two energies in each of his hands and seen what those hands did. I would also have worked more openly on this issue with the family and talked to them about how they could work with both being such powerful people who were dedicated to everyone being so close and with working things out.

In contrast, the first woman I ever worked with in a coma, Josie, had a very different kind of response from her children. One of her daughters had told me that she hoped her mother would die and that it wouldn't be much of a loss. She was sitting at her mother's bedside when she said this, and her mother jerked so intensely that she almost sat up in bed. We repeated this experience several times. I was at my limits of my experience and training at that time. Now I would have gone back and done family therapy right over the bed. I would have spoken for the mother and taken her side in the conflict with the daughters. I would have played out the ghost roles of hatred and dismissal that this whole experience was calling up, and then I would have supported the mother's reaction even more. From my own center, I would have helped these sides to get to know each other more—one side that seemed to say something like "love me" and the other side that said something like "I hate you." I am sure that these roles were in both the daughters and the mother, so I would have helped the roles to express themselves more fluidly so that the mother could bring out her hatred in response, and maybe the daughters could have brought in some of the original pain and need that they had before they became so hard toward the mother. The feelings that had always been around toward the mother were being expressed more clearly now that she was in a coma. Her other daughters wanted their mother to be able to recover, and felt very sad about her condition. They were working hard to help her come back; however, this one daughter had always felt neglected by her mother who had always favored the other daughters and been cold toward her. The daughter was reflecting that coldness back to her mother while she was in the coma. Maybe for the first time, the daughter felt safe enough to bring these feelings forward. Maybe coma is meant to open doors for individuals to go where they have never gone, and possibly could never go while in a state of ordinary consciousness. Maybe coma is meant to do the same thing for this and other families, to amplify and to dramatically express what has been in the background forever, in the hopes that facing things might make them more fluid.

In another family, there was an issue with the father, Herman, around how unemotional he had been as a parent. He was in a coma, and during this time the family began to explore their own feelings about one another and in relation to their father. Herman had been given no chance of survival or recovery by his doctors. However, one evening, after a very emotional afternoon of processing with the family, I told him about what we had been doing and he began to cry. Within an hour-and-a-half, he was speaking, and then came fully out of the coma. He was much more feeling in his interactions with people after this coma.

The family felt the coma had facilitated them working on this issue. The family needed to get to the edge of life and death to work on their issues openly and to let their own emotions fly and be processed. Herman reflected their own frozenness, but the situation was so tense and extreme that the family stepped into their emotions, and then Herman could step into his and follow his feelings back to being more fully conscious.

On another occasion I was being driven to the hospital by Lennie, who was going to see his brother Jack for the first time since his heart attack. We talked about how tragic it had been for the family. Then Lennie said something that stunned me. He said it might also be more useful for the family as everyone seemed to be doing better since Jack had gone into the coma. Apparently this dislike had been in the background for many years. Lennie told me that his brother had been a tyrant who dominated everyone at home and at the family business. Jack was critical, driven, and drove everyone. When he had his heart attack, everyone suddenly felt like a dictator had fallen, and they were free. I wonder what effect this level of background dislike had on Jack's heart and on the fact that he'd had a heart attack. My own idea is that nothing just happens out of nowhere. Jack had attacked everyone in the family for years, and probably attacked himself, too. He may never have acknowledged it, but his own heart had for sure felt all of the feelings of hatred and revenge his family had for him. If we could take a psychic picture or X-ray of his heart, I would expect to see something like a war zone of unprocessed agony that had been there forever before his heart "attacked him." Several years ago, the psychologist and spiritual teacher Ram Dass said in a talk I heard in Eugene, Oregon, that he didn't have a stroke, he had been stroked. The stroke was a process he somehow needed, that slowed him down and made him even more present. Jack didn't have a heart attack, his heart attacked him; in the coma, he was able to let all that rage out that seemed to just be seething in the background and turning everyone against him for reasons he could probably never understand.

When this family interacted with Jack in coma, the interactions looked radically different from those of Sandy's family who stayed by his side every moment. In the three examples, we had a family who just loved the person as their interaction, a family that was motivated to work deeply on emotional issues, and a family that rejected the patient. These are just a few of the deep family processes that come up and can be engaged with using a Process-oriented approach to working with families dealing with a coma.

In yet another story, a father, Victor, had had a stroke and ended up in a coma. This experience clarified to the family that a key issue they had been struggling with was having free time together. Victor was in the restaurant business and worked around the clock. Now, in the coma, he was on vacation, but in a most unrelated way. The whole work with this family was around the issues of dad and his overwork. The family's theory was that overworking had caused the stroke, and now, in the coma, their father could rest. Of course now looking back, I have bigger questions I would have explored, such as how to help these two energies of nonstop work and vacation work it out with each other. This comes again from the essence work and Earth-based work that emphasizes the relationship between the conflicting sides present in symptoms. Saying yes to the work side, and yes to the vacation side, I would have said: "So, dear Victor, is there any way to work out this internal struggle besides balancing your work with a coma?" Maybe not, but maybe a different arrangement might have made the coma state unnecessary.

These four examples are all about working with the personal issues of the family member in the coma—Sandy's anger, Josie's coldness, Herman's lack of emotional expression, and Jack's dominant nature—although these intrapersonal issues also impacted on the whole family. Yet these were clearly also family issues. If the individual was working with these tensions, then the family had probably not only struggled with these tensions during their lifetime but possibly over many generations.

In other cases a coma may amplify interpersonal issues more directly. In one family, where the son was in a coma, the marital problems of the parents that had led to divorce came to the foreground. The parents had radically different belief systems about life and its meaning, and they fought over whether or not I could work with their son. The father believed that coma was a physical state, and that beyond medical inter-vention, not much could be done. The mother believed that coma was meaningful and that her son could be reached. These differences had always existed between mom and dad. But their son's coma brought these philosophical battles to the foreground. Mom was much more grounded in her spiritual view toward life, and dad was more grounded in the world of day-by-day consensus reality. Dad followed the medical view and believed that all that could be done was loving, physical care. Mom believed in every possible alternative therapy, including all kinds of spir-itual methods. With our support and facilitation, each of them was able to follow their views of life, and brought out their love for their son based on this worldview. In this way, I was doing more Earth-based work, allowing these polarities to come forward, for each to be supported, and to get to know each other and find ways of working together rather than against each other. Was that a coma—yes—and was it also a way of bringing together these polarized aspects of the family to work with each other? My answer for sure is—yes. The parents were divorced, but the coma allowed, even necessitated, the polarization to work on itself so that they could come up with a treatment program for their child.

In another family I worked with, the split was just the opposite. The mom was totally connected to her son's medical care and believed this was all that could be done, while the dad brought in alternative practitioners from all over the world. Then the two of them would fight over the practitioners, arguing about which of us was helpful and not, and other related issues. With what I know now, I would have seen this as two sides getting to know each other, and I would have encouraged them to work on learning about each other's side and to recognize its value. I would know that having them not only work on this polarity that was incredibly relevant to working out the medical care for their son, but also that these two positions being so at odds must be related to the son's coma. Everyone in a family works together on the same ancient polarities that have always plagued the family, and the coma gives the family a highly motivational situation to work on these differences.

In other coma cases the whole family struggles may also be amplified and need to be worked on. In one family, Fred was in coma. His wife had pushed her stepdaughters further and further out of the picture. One of the most dramatic moments I remember was one of the daughters coming in from college to be with her father, and she and her stepmother reconciling and embracing right over Fred's bed. The family had a belief that part of what Fred was doing in the coma was escaping the horrible level of alienation and conflict between the family members, particularly between different family factions. Step-sibling rivalry, tension between the stepmother and children, and the tensions between the ex-wife and the current wife had turned the family into a war zone. Process-oriented Coma Work in this situation involved simultaneously working on the man in the coma, and working on processing these family tensions.

So in summary, it is important to work on all the different levels in a family when someone is in coma. The work may focus either on an individual and their growth, on a relationship dynamic between people, or on issues relating to the whole family system. This is the same theory we have in group and large group work in Process-oriented work. We say that it is important to identify the level at which we are working: individual focus, relationship, group, or the world. The same thing applies to families, and in fact, sometimes the family work focuses on the world. I remember once working on a young woman who was in a coma after having been blown up by a terrorist attack. I couldn't work on her without bringing up all the politics of experience that were involved with all of this. I asked her whether, if we could do something about the horrible violence between the sides, it would make it easier for her to come out of coma.

My own belief is that not only does the family benefit from clearing up issues, but that it has a positive effect on the person in the coma, too. Often the issues that need to be addressed directly with the person in the coma were also present before the coma. I remember standing over the bedside of one woman in coma and noticing how distant her husband was. I recommended that he stroke his wife's face and give her a kiss. He had tremendous resistance to doing this, but was eventually able to, and his wife seemed to smile when he kissed her. The next morning she came out of the coma. I don't think this was just a coincidence; relationship for some people is a matter of life and death. When she came out of the coma, this woman talked to me in detail about her issues around her husband's distance and how depressing the lack of physical contact had been. I have found in my own research that there has almost always been a major source of depression present before a coma, even if the coma involves something like an auto accident. It is important to work directly on these sources of depression even while the person is in a coma.

DEALING WITH MIXED EMOTIONS IN FAMILIES WITH COMA

The entire spectrum of human emotions shows up when a family member is in a coma. Some of the most common feelings present are shock, grief, sadness, despair, depression, anger, guilt, and remorse. Much of the anger is often directed at the hospital, which sometimes deserves it for being insensitive to the needs of coma patients and their loved ones. In addition, the hospital may also serve as an outlet for the incredible frustrations people feel in relation to coma. I consider most of these feelings to be related to attachment. Attachment in this context means that I, as a family member, want to hold on to my loved one and have them come back to me the way they used to be. I am usually convinced that not enough is being done for them, otherwise if it were they would get better and come out of this coma. I won't accept anything less than full recovery, and usually I am connected to this goal, so I can't easily relate to or accept where the person is now, in this comatose state. These feelings are usually in the foreground, and they need facilitation to be fully expressed. I have worked with many families who, because of their focus on recovery, have never felt free to shed a tear for their loved one in the coma, or have never been able to get angry at the person who caused the automobile accident that left their loved one in a coma.

Sensitive family therapists need to be prepared to utilize all of their facilitation skills to help the family come to grips with the emotions that emerge. Families often tend to polarize around two roles: being in total despair and giving up all hope or being in total denial and being sure that although the person hasn't given any feedback in two years, they will wake up at any moment. The family therapist may at times need to help families in both directions—supporting both their despair and their optimism and helping them come to a more realistic assessment of the situation.

Sometimes families must make life and death decisions and they need to be able to make realistic assessments. Some of the possible decisions they may need to make include whether life support systems should be applied or held back, the degree of resuscitation that should be utilized if the person stops breathing, what kind of surgery can be attempted, and other similar decisions of awesome responsibility. At moments like this, it is helpful if therapists have both family therapy and Process-oriented Coma Work skills, and are also willing to dialogue with medical professionals. From a Process-oriented standpoint, there is a lot of hope for coma patients, but there is also the reality that people in certain kinds of comas have a greater likelihood of coming out than people in other kinds of comas. Of course the type of coma, the extent of brain damage, the amount of time without oxygen, and all of these other consensus reality factors influence the prognosis, but a prognosis is just a prediction; life and death decisions need to reflect the reality that a prognosis isn't a death sentence.

Therapists and family members in a coma situation face a uniquely challenging scenario. When someone dies, the family has something painful but definitive to face. When someone is ill, the medical staff can usually give a fairly accurate prognosis. Unfortunately in coma, although there is some level of predictability based on the factors mentioned above, there is also a great deal of unpredictability and much of the time there is simply no way to know what will happen. Time and nature work their course, and in some cases people come out of comas even though medical opinion considered their chances of awakening to be nonexistent.

Having a family member in a coma gives the family and their therapist an incredible opportunity to explore their reactions to the unknown aspects of life and death. In the "information age" we live in, facing the unknown can be a rare, terrifying, and potentially enlightening experience.

In this realm, many people who have never identified themselves as spiritual suddenly experience a deepening of their connection with some eternal presence, whether they identify this as God, nature, Buddha, Christ, the Great Spirit, or some other manifestation of divine connection. Other people rely more on their human relationships to pull them through such difficult times. Most people seem to rely on both human and divine connections to face such times of unknowing.

The more families experience their emotions and experience the unknown, the more a second series of feelings come up. I put these feelings under the complementary heading of detachment. By detachment I mean being able to let go of expectations and meeting the person in coma in the here and now, as they are. It may also mean accepting death as part of life, or accepting that the person may never be the same as they were before the coma. Detachment can also mean releasing ourselves from the guilt, or the obligations of visiting as much, or even of being with the person at all. Frequently people start to feel that the connection with the person isn't physical, rather it is maintained through their feelings or their dreams about the person. People start to accept more where the person is at and accept their relationship as it is, instead of staying stuck in their need for the situation to change. Many families are more reticent about their feelings of detachment than about the grief, loss, anger, and frustration that they experience, and feelings of detachment need to be supported as much as the feelings of grief, loss, and anger.

Family members of someone in a coma may spend months just sitting in a hospital, sometimes without seeing any major changes in their loved one. Even in cases where the family members are attached and totally love the person in the coma, moments of letting go arise. Letting go is a survival mechanism; eventually we must all move on and take care of ourselves. This may mean momentarily leaving a loved one behind. In cultures that support feelings of detachment, for example, in Buddhist-based cultures, where letting go and being free from attachment to material concerns is a part of their everyday philosophy, getting families to identify with their detachment is not as difficult as it is in Western cultures, where the medical and philosophical systems are based on saving people. In certain Buddhist teachings and cultures, for example, in Zen Buddhism, death is meditated on from a young age. It is a part of life, and so, unlike in the West, it is not viewed as a medical failure if someone dies, but rather as a normal part of moving on through many lifetimes. From this detached point of view, holding on to a particular lifetime for too long might be seen as impairing the flow of development that may take many, many lifetimes.

In my experience, families usually need help with two major kinds of letting go. First of all, as families process all of their feelings, they may experience more moments where they simply need some relief and permission to focus on other parts of life. I recently worked with an extremely dedicated family, where the parents really needed support to take some vacation time and also some couple time together. After about six months of being with their son without a break, they were able to go away for a weekend together. Many times this letting go is enough—people just need short breaks, maybe even encouragement to let themselves have a night off will be enough.

The other type of letting go is more challenging and may mean allowing the person in the coma to die. In this case letting go may involve dropping attachment to the person in the coma waking up. Process-oriented Coma Work helps with this because it helps family members connect and have a relationship with the person in the coma. For many people, they can't let go if they can't connect first. Letting go is a very intimate, personal matter. I remember the last time I was with my father, the way I touched and held his hands as he was dying. I loved him so much and loved his hands and held those hands. We had such an intimate time together. I drove off with my partner Sage and burst into tears, knowing that by connecting with him physically, I could let go of our physical connection. I never have let go of our emotional or spiritual connection, but I knew that was the end of our being able to be physically in touch.

Janice, whose son was in a coma, told me that she felt the closest she had ever felt to him while he was in the coma. She felt that the essence of who her son was felt closer to the surface then before. She could just feel his incredibly sweet and loving nature, and this allowed her to bring hers out more with him. Their love flowed back and forth in ways that it hadn't when both of them had been more contained with their feelings toward each other, as that was the way teens and parents are "supposed to be with each other," according to culture. This is an example of Janice being able to let go of the past relationship and value and flow with the current coma-based relationship with her son.

Letting go at other points might mean putting less emphasis on the person in coma and moving back into taking care of one's own health, career, or relationship. Or it may mean letting go of guilt to feel okay about spending less time with the person in coma. For some people, it may mean letting them eventually have a new best friend or a new lover, knowing that the person in a coma may never be available again. I have watched many cases where people have eventually moved on to a new love. This is complicated emotionally, since the person in the coma may someday come out. The family therapist is in the role of the ally to the family's wholeness, letting them know that all feelings of attachment and detachment are normal and need to be explored and expressed.

THE FAMILY AS A MIRROR OF THE PERSON IN THE COMA

From my own observation and from talking to other coma workers, it seems that the way the family feels about an individual in coma may not only reflect the feelings of individual family members and a collective feeling toward the person in coma, but may also mirror the feelings of the person in coma. The long-term level of enthusiasm of the family members for staying with the person in coma seems to reflect the interest level of the person in the coma. Some people I work with in coma are interactive and give a lot of feedback. Others are difficult to contact and show little interest in interacting and especially not in waking up, while still others seem to be struggling to wake up with all of their strength. Family attitudes seem to parallel the situation of the person in the coma.

One family I worked with seemed to have very little interest in their mother who was in a coma. When she first went into a coma, the interest level of a few members was high, but within a few months, no one showed much interest. She was in a nursing home, lying in bed by herself most days. Her reaction to me was very similar to the family's attitude. She seemed disinterested in working with me. I would drive quite a distance to see her, and after hours of work, have almost no feedback. In contrast, I once worked with a man where the two women who loved him most, his wife and a close friend, were always at his side along with his other friends. Even after a year in coma, the man showed so much interest in the work that he was able to communicate with us by wiggling his finger for yes and no answers, and at one point he started to vibrate so much that he almost jumped out of the bed. It was so dramatic that we were all in tears.

Based on these observations, I have added a new step to my assessment of the chances of the person coming out of the coma. In addition to looking at medical records, checking for feedback, and consulting with other professionals, I also study in great detail the level of interest of family members. This interest level could be explained partially by the signals of the client, that is, a client who gives lots of feedback will help hold family members' interest; however, there is something more mystical and unexplainable beyond this. The family seems to pull back before the coma patient pulls away, and family member interest seems to have a resurgence before coma patients get better. Maybe there is something deeply instinctual about this—similar to the way animals leave a dying animal alone. They know for their survival they must move on. Possibly this is more evidence that we are in non-local contact always with each other, and possibly this is even more true with coma patients. There is some deep kind of communication that is not only signal-based, but people constantly feel and dream about the person in coma. Maybe we also receive their signals to come closer, or to let them be, as well as their signals to join them in fighting for life and recovery, or letting them be so as to allow them to stay in the coma or die. Of course, at times letting them be is just what they also need to help them come out; however, what I am trying to describe is a feeling experience between coma and loved one. For example, in my father's case, his medical team told me when they thought my Dad would die. I told them no, he would die a few weeks later, and he did. I felt it; there was some kind of irrational knowing. I stuck with my intuition and timed my visit based on this, to say goodbye, but it was difficult coming from a family of doctors all telling me he would not still be alive.

COMA AS A ROLE IN THE FAMILY

The person in coma carries a particular spot in the family system. They often are closest to the most forbidden parts of family life. They are in altered and extreme states, not related to the outer world, deeply internal. Especially at the beginning of the coma, they receive tremendous amounts of care, focus, and attention.

One important exercise for a family to try is to have everyone temporarily become more like the person in a coma. It is important to ask all family members about their own tendencies toward extreme states and to help them go into these extreme states consciously. For example, having the whole family sit quietly, go inside, and then describe their experiences can be very powerful.

The most powerful intervention I know is to have the family members lie down and pretend that they are in a coma. With the assistance of someone trained in Coma Work, family members go through the kinds of feeling, visual, auditory, and movement experiences that come up as they imagine themselves in this state. This usually produces important and deep experiences. I recently did this with a family and their friends who are working closely with the person in coma. The whole support team went down into the coma state. Some felt quiet, while others felt very emotional. One person had been terrified of getting lost, but she had a good experience just going inside herself. Another found it hard to give up control long enough to go into this state, but when she did, she got in touch with her need to rest. All the people I have done this with have said that they benefited, in that they felt closer to the experience the coma person was having. Their ways of working with the person also became more sensitive. Most had a positive experience and began to realize that not all experiences a coma person is having are negative. Some got in touch with parts of themselves they were not aware of before.

In theory at least, this intervention should also be helpful to the person in a coma. Systems theory suggests that if the whole system picks up a role or way of being that the identified patient has been carrying alone, it should help relieve the symptoms of the individual. I have seen this happen many times when someone in a group is in an extreme state. When the group picks this up, the person may temporarily leave the extreme state and take up the "normal" role.

The other reason this role switch from caregiver to the one in need of care is so important is because of the burnout issue. I address these issues in detail in Chapter 7. Taking care of any family member or friend who is ill over a long period of time can exhaust a whole family. Giving care is an important role, but it is not all of life. Caregivers also need lots of care, but when a crisis occurs, most family members forget about themselves and just focus on the other. By playing the role of the one who needs care, people can remember their own needs. The family members need to take care of themselves not only for their own sake, but also for the sake of being able to provide long-term care for the patient. One dramatic way to do this switching exercise, in a relaxed setting such as when a patient is at home, is to ask people to try lying down on the bed next to the patient and see what it is like to be the one who needs care, or even just to do this in their imagination.

Finally, it may be important to work on family issues directly with the person in coma. For example, I told one young man, Jeremy, that I would help him find his way in his career if he came out, even to the extent of supporting him to explore jobs that might go against the family traditions. I told another person that I would help with all the family conflicts now and continue to do so if he came out, and that he did not need to stay in the coma just to avoid these terrible conflicts. I have also said to people that they should feel free to follow their own processes around living and dying, coming out and not coming out, rather than just reacting to family pressure. And I've also had family members talk directly to the person in coma, telling them what was in their hearts that might be relevant to the person staying in or coming out of coma.

On one level coma looks like a unique state that has nothing to do with ordinary family interactions. Yet it is important to learn about relating to people in comatose states for several reasons. First, many of us will have loved ones who spend time in a coma. Second, much of what happens in the roles, feelings, and issues that come up in Coma

Work is no different than what happens in ordinary states of consciousness. When we are not in a coma, sometimes we want to relate and other times not. Although people in comas generally don't relate in ordinary ways, they are also sometimes very related, and other times not. Also, family members often get locked into roles. For example, one is always the caring one, another is the good child, another is the one in trouble. One way to view the comatose person is to see that they are locked into a role that needs to be worked on within the family. Comas provide a creative opportunity for working on relationships between the family and person in the coma and between other family members. Third, the sensitivity that is involved in relating to someone in coma can also help us in other relationships. In my coma classes, I often joke that if you want to become the most sensitive lover, spend time trying to relate to someone in a coma. Comatose people are the best teachers on picking up feedback, a skill that helps us learn to be great lovers.

COMA, FAMILIES, AND NON-LOCALITY

In Process Work we talk of the family as being a field. We are affected not only by what happens directly but also by the atmosphere around us. Arnold Mindell's *Sitting in the Fire* defines the field as "the atmosphere or climate of any community, including its physical, environmental, and emotional surroundings."[1] Families are like a community. What happens with one member, or any part of a family, may affect the whole family even if they aren't all physically present. We see this in Coma Work, when we work on family issues in another room and then a major shift happens to the person in coma. We don't just have to wait for this kind of field effect to happen, we can consciously do family work to see how it moves the person. While working in another part of the country, I saw one young person who was in a coma whose parents told me that she had started to develop all kinds of physical symptoms, had accidents, and made suicide attempts at a time when they were experiencing very painful periods in their marriage. Although it was important to work with the young person and to move her arms and legs and work with her eye movements and all the normal signal work I do, the family problem was also described as part of the symptom. It was in the field, the palatable family atmosphere, so that this client could feel and almost breathe in the marital tensions in her own body. So I told the parents we should also work on their marital issues that they had never addressed. They were quite hopeless about this, maybe even more hopeless about this than the young person's recovery, but agreed to do it for the sake of their young one, Jenelle. Who was in coma—Jenelle, the relationship, or both? Also, their region and their country as a whole seemed to be in a coma, unable to respond to the ongoing problems, trauma, and challenges of the times. The whole Coma Work then became research into whether it would affect Janelle if this couple's relationship changes and they come out of their "coma." Jenelle. Also, if they don't change, how might this affect the coma? How many people might wake up out of coma if the whole planet were more awake and conscious of its issues of war, ecology, race, economics, and so many other central issues? These are research questions I am exploring together with my colleagues worldwide. My experience, though, has been that we are all connected, and working on a system or any part of a system moves that system. A really simple example of this is how often in my private practice clients will tell me that after they worked on a family issue, suddenly that family member who hasn't called for years suddenly calls, or another family member acts completely differently. Our family connections are definitely non-local and, in my personal experience, not only transcend location but also time and life and death itself. Many of my clients report visitations or communications with their loved ones who have died. When I hear this from someone who is mystical and believes in these kinds of things, it is not so impressive, but when I hear this over and over again from my more mainstream clients, it makes me think we are so much more connected than we ever imagined. If we could really know and experience this, our own death and the deaths of our loved ones would still be painful but possibly not so scary.

To help you explore these issues, here are two exercises (Exercises 4.1 and 4.2) that I designed to help us understand how family patterns might affect comatose states. All of us have had certain states of consciousness that we marginalized due to family and cultural expectations.

One aspect of our family work is to be a bridge between what the family is experiencing and the medical model. Families may notice very small shifts in consciousness but the medical system only recognizes major shifts. In the case I have previously mentioned, where Herman recuperated fully from a stroke, the head neurologist, who was also a neurosurgeon, said that he didn't consider the fact that Herman could talk again to be a really significant shift as he wasn't yet speaking three sentences in a row. Eventually he admitted that moving from being ready to pull life support to talking at all was something. The coma worker, without giving the family false hope, can support the real changes present and give them encouragement to continue to do what they are doing that works. The coma worker can point out

Exercise 4.1
Childhood Experiences and Comas

Part 1

1.	What state do you still long for that, since childhood, you have never felt you could quite get to or get enough of?
2.	Now imagine you were in a state of minimal responsiveness, coming out of coma, where you could be in this state all the time. What would this world be like?
3.	How have you noticed that world you long for calling you recently? How is it present in your dreams, body symptoms, relationship issues, and world challenges?

Part 2

4.	Next, with four people and a facilitator, re-create your family system; tell people how to be like your family.
5.	Now go into this comatose state you so long for and stay there.
6.	The job of the facilitator is to create a link between the family and the person in this state, and to try and help the family to meet and address some of the deepest needs of the person in coma. The family could experiment with working on some of its issues and see how this affects the person in coma.
7.	After 20 minutes, give the facilitator feedback and switch.

Exercise 4.2
Family Work and Movement
The purpose of this exercise is to have the whole family become the secondary state of the patient and then work with sentient movement.

---

1. Have the family agree on a definition of what it is in the client's state that is most different from the rest of the family. For example, Suzy is quieter than the rest of us, or Fred is not as productive as every one else, or Mohammed is wilder than we are, etc. Ask the family to make up a dream figure that represents this energy. Maybe their loved one is a Buddha, or a whale in the ocean, or a bird flying, or whatever seems appropriate.
2. Ask the family to discover the deepest characteristic of this dream figure and name it.
3. Have all of the family then play out and be this essence. For example, if the dream figure is Buddha and the essence is quiet stillness, all the family will be this.
4. Now have the family all close their eyes, in the same area as the coma person, and each person should slowly follow their inner movement, their impulses, and see what happens.
5. Ask afterward how what happened may be a key to the coma person taking the next step, whatever that may be.

---

denial of hope in either direction—false hopes and premature letting go of hope.

It is very helpful to do either direct or indirect family therapy with the family present. Direct would be a formal family session. I ask the family if they would rather do this privately or in the room with the person in coma. Sometimes issues specifically related to the person in coma are processed, like a fight over a divorce or what have you. Sometimes it is other longstanding family issues. At other times it is more like working with the ghost roles and the spirits present in the family, and seeing how the extreme state of the person in coma is representative of something the whole family somehow needs. Ghost roles and family spirits here refer to the hidden, unspoken, yet clearly felt, unidentified roles and energies present. Showing these roles and playing them out is often helpful. For example, in a family where the ghost role is someone who is very sensual and loves physical contact, then playing this out with the person in coma, or with each other, might be very healing for the whole family system.

RELATIONSHIP STYLES AND COMA WORK

I began this chapter by talking about the four kinds of attitudes toward relationship with people in comas. To review, these are:

1. Being interested in relationship before coma and in coma.
2. Being interested before coma, but not in coma.
3. Being disinterested before coma and interested during coma.
4. Being disinterested before and during coma.

I will now illustrate each of these types with case studies. These cases are based on reports from family members of how the person was before and during coma, and on my own observations.

In terms of the first type of person, related before and during the coma, there are two categories within this larger category. The first is the person who has negative relationships before the coma and during, but is very involved in the relationships in both states. The person I think of to illustrate is Jack who had had a heart attack and who everyone seemed to hate. He wasn't very good at relationship before coma and was always in relationship trouble, so he spent lots of time relating, even if it was negative in its effects. He was also totally related in the coma and wanted to fight and fight. His style in coma was similar to out of coma. I have included this example because it illustrates that by relating I mean being involved in relationships, whether in negative or positive ways.

The next case demonstrates being interested in relationships in a positive way before and during coma. I call her Nina. She lived in the Midwest, and I had known her from various different groups we both belonged to. She was always involved with people. She worked with people, was a social activist involved with people, engaged with her family and friends, and in her spare time helped those less fortunate than herself. I was called in to work with her when she had gone into coma from a brain tumor. When I remember our session together, I still get goose bumps. She was lying in a room where everyone thought she should be quiet. She was at the hospital, and people thought she needed to be left alone with pretty music and lots of rest. I noticed that she wasn't very interested in all this rest, so I started to interact with her in a very energetic way. Initially her family and friends needed reassuring, as they thought I might hurt her if she didn't just rest, but there wasn't anything in her medical condition that said interaction would be harmful. She loved the stimulation. At one point I started to tell her what a hot, intense, lovely woman she was, and at that moment the nurses ran through the unit and shut all the room doors including ours. A fire alarm had gone off at the moment I was saying how hot she was. These kinds of synchronistic experiences are a common occurrence when working with coma patients and are part of what convinces me that we are tapping into deeply rooted places in the person's being. It turned out the fire alarm was a false alarm, but it encouraged me to go further with her hot nature. I told her husband to give her a big kiss on the lips. He looked at me like I was crazy, but eventually gave it a try. She responded by puckering up to meet his lips, and when he stopped she kept puckering as if to ask for more. The next morning, she woke up out of her coma.

The second style, being related before the coma but not during, is best illustrated by Irene, a woman I worked with briefly who was the epitome of relationship before the coma. She was described by her family as the perfect mother, always present first for her children and then her grandchildren. Irene lived on a farm, where she took constant excellent care of her animals. In the coma, she looked relaxed, happy, and totally disinterested in relationship. The family members had said that before the coma she had been planning to go on a long vacation. It looks like Irene found her long vacation by having a stroke and being in the coma. Perhaps she couldn't get the break she needed from people while being in an ordinary state of consciousness. Since she lived far away from where I live, I was only able to spend a few hours with her, but I have never, before or since, seen someone who looked so congruently happy in a coma, and so totally disinterested in the outer world of people and events.

Louie was from France. He illustrates a different version of being related before the coma and both unrelated and related during the coma. He has very selective relatedness. He was the best example of selective relationship attention in coma that I have ever had. Louie had been in a coma from an auto accident, and at the one year mark was given no chance of improvement of any kind. He had a very close family who were constantly talking to him, touching him, and spending lots of time literally right in his face, a few inches from his face. Louie went further and further away, deeper and deeper into coma the more they related to him. He was described as a very nice young man before coma, very loving and connected with his family and others. However, another pattern became evident during the Coma Work. Louie had gone to school far away from his parents. He was also far away from them in coma. I had a very difficult time connecting with Louie. One day his wonderful girlfriend showed up, and Louie seemed totally interested. I saw him do something that still gives me a bit of a shock. She came over to him, and he put his hand right under her blouse and touched her breast. It was obvious she wasn't wearing a bra, and that Louie was interested in not only connecting with her personality but with her breasts. He wouldn't touch anyone else, but he would touch her sensually. The strongest intervention that I ever made was to ask the family to leave the two of them alone. The family was very resistive, but eventually gave them alone time. She told me afterward that Louie had gone much further and touched her much more sexually, and she had found ways to respond. Louie seemed much more present the next day, and although he was still head injured and had a long way to go, that was his turning point in terms of his recovery. I heard that several years later, he was still living with his girlfriend in a supported living apartment for people with head injuries, and he was doing well except with speech.

Herman's case illustrates the third type of being unrelated before the coma, and related in the coma. I talked in detail earlier about Herman who had had a stroke and was going to be removed from life support, but came back when I was telling him about his family working on their issues. He had been very unrelated before coma, but during and after coma, made all of his breakthroughs in the relationship realms. Once out of coma he told me his motivation was to be present and work out his issues with his family. Coma was the vehicle of transformation for him from unrelated to taking relationship seriously. Would he have made this transformation without the coma? I am not sure as his life seemed headed in such a different direction. The coma seemed to be the most rapid and direct way of changing

Louise's case illustrates the fourth type of being unrelated in life and in coma. Louise had been a successful professional in life, but was severely

depressed and withdrawn. Her own relationship life was limited to interacting with a few family members. She is one of many whom I have
worked with who worked in the medical profession, and although dedicat-
ing her life to working with people, had little relationship life of her own.
When I worked with her, her family tried so hard to get her to connect
with them, but she seemed so disinterested. Although we had momentary
breakthroughs, she seemed particularly unrelated. I wasn't able to work
with her for more than a day, but the family said she was more related that
day than most. I was able to help other therapists work with her, but they
focused much more on helping her with her internal states than her relationship life. Either this wasn't the channel that was working for her, or
her lack of relatedness was something we couldn't find our way around
while working with her in the coma. Again I only had one day with her,
and I am not sure what would have happened over many days of working.

Finally, I want to talk about Helen, who demonstrated to me how
powerful relationship can be during coma. She doesn't easily fit into any
category. Helen had been on dialysis for years, and decided at a certain
point to stop, knowing this would mean she would first go into a coma
and then die. Even before she did this, she had decided to confront and
clean up all kinds of relationship issues in her life, including telling off a
pastor who she felt had put her down and made her feel guilty and horrible about who she was. She worked it out with family, friends, and with
clergy so that by the time she was ready to die she was ready to go. I
worked with her as she was going into her altered states before coma, and
then I had to leave town. I kept thinking about her during the day while I
was teaching in another city, and decided to give her a call. The nurse
answered and said that she was in a deep coma and was moments from
death. She hadn't related to anyone in many days. I asked the nurse to put
the phone up to her ear, and I said "Helen, it's Gary. I just wanted to tell
you to have a good journey home." I also told her how much I loved her.
Suddenly she said to me, "Gary, I love you, too." I asked her how she was
and she replied "Gary, I couldn't be better." We talked a bit more, and then
I told her I had to go back to teaching. The nurse was stunned, as Helen
hadn't spoken for days. When I called back, they said Helen had died 12
minutes after we spoke. Maybe she was waiting for that phone call, but she
had the power to come out of coma to say good-bye.

RELATIONSHIP CRISIS AND COMA

I have worked with several people who went into a coma immediately
after a major relationship conflict or painful moment. One was a man

named Leonard, whom I worked with outside the United States. He had a heart attack the day after his relationship partner had told him she didn't really love him. He was an older man, and after this heart attack, he never recovered fully. During the Coma Work, he responded well to his partner telling him that she had made a terrible mistake and she totally loved him. The coma state allowed her to take care of him and show him how much she really loved him. They had many close and related moments during the Coma Work, as he would respond to her by turning his head, moving his mouth, and showing other signals that he would show only with her.

In another case, I worked with a young man here in the United States who had a stroke the moment after his wife told him that she wouldn't have sex with him. He immediately became agitated and had a stroke. He came out of the coma enough to speak while we worked with him, and is still in a long rehabilitation process.

Finally, one time we worked on a man in a coma where I had a dream about him. I woke up having had a dream about someone in trouble for having an affair. A few minutes later, at about 6:30 A.M., the phone rang. His wife called and asked me to meet her for coffee before we worked on her husband. She said that her husband had a stroke while traveling. She thought he was traveling for work. When she found out about the stroke, she called his work to find out the details, and it turned out the trip wasn't about work. He was seeing another woman with whom he'd had a secret life; he'd had an ongoing affair for years with separate bank accounts for their relationship and other hidden features. The stroke brought this whole affair to light, as the wife found the other woman at her husband's hospital bedside and the whole truth had come out.

Was the coma in some way meant to reveal all of this truth that the husband wasn't able to directly reveal? We can only speculate. We helped his wife process all of her feelings about this with her husband in one of the most intense relationship works I have ever done as a coma therapist. As she expressed her feelings, he began to wiggle and turn away, and she wouldn't let him. She turned him back and made him listen. She said without doing this and clearing some of her feelings with him directly, she couldn't go on caring for him. She was looking after him in their bedroom at home, in a hospital bed, where she might have to care for him for years, and she needed the emotional clearing. He also seemed more alert after this. We lost touch with this woman after several months and I am not sure how far back he ever came.

All of these cases with relationship and coma where the reactions are so extreme raise many different questions that we can explore. My own theory is that if we can process hurt and rejection and we know how to do this, our system doesn't experience the level of shock that these experiences bring. Saying someone broke someone's heart seems to be quite literal for some of my patients. There are two major ways I see Process Work helping to prevent this kind of blow to our system. First, Arnold Mindell has said repeatedly over the years that major developments in our lives do not just come out of nowhere. No partner just gets up and leaves us without some kind of signal or trail of signals. Noticing these signals allows us to possibly address the issues that are trying to come forward, which may prevent a break up or make it something that is more mutual and less of a shock. Once the moment of break up or sexual rejection comes up, if we know methods like Process Work, we allow ourselves to go into the feelings of shock and feel them, but then we also go beyond the shock and process our hurt and anger in a way that helps us to clear those emotions. If I can really listen to my heart and follow it closely, there is less chance that it will attack me and I will have a heart attack. If I allow my brain to go into altered states around relationships, there is less chance of a stroke or other extreme phenomena in my brain. It is like being a runner. If I am trained as a runner and I suddenly have to run when someone chases me, it is less likely I will get injured than if I haven't exercised for a long time and I suddenly have to run for my life. The Tibetan Buddhists say we need to train for living and for dying, to be prepared. I share this view.

Pierre: Gary eloquently described many relationship aspects of our work with comatose clients and their families. I will now expand on some of the relationship aspects that will come up in the work with people who have come out of their coma and are confronted with changes in their sense of self and identity. The example I am presenting is about someone who is coping with internalized relationship conflicts between his old and new self and the external conflicts that are caused by changes in his personality.

I am currently counseling Chris, a young man, husband, and father of a three-year-old girl. Almost a year ago he had an accident on his bicycle. He was going for a small errand and took his bike. Apparently, the doctor told him, his left lung spontaneously collapsed (a rare case in some tall white men with high lung capacity where the pleura has thin spots that can collapse spontaneously). He was riding downhill and hit a truck. His head didn't hit anything but spun around and then brutally stopped. The acceleration and sudden stop of the brain inside the scull led to a diffuse axonal injury, a shearing of the nerves. Chris describes it as an insane accident that happened out of the blue caused by an act of a higher power or God. His doctors told him he was extremely lucky that he didn't break his neck or fracture his skull. It was a miracle accident and a miracle survival.

In his counseling with me I asked him to tell me about an early childhood dream or memory. In what way, you might ask, is one's childhood dream of any relevance in the rehabilitation process after coma? The association comes from the work of C.G. Jung, who, between 1936 and 1941, taught four seminars on children's dreams (these seminars have recently been published in English). In his introductory remarks, Jung makes this interesting observation: "These early dreams in particular are of utmost importance because they are dreamed out of the depth of personality and, therefore, frequently represent an anticipation of the later destiny."[2] So it seems that childhood dreams or early memories often contain the themes and patterns that guide our adult lives and personal development or *individuation*. Knowledge of such memories can help us put certain experiences in a personal context and help us find meaning in what seem to be random events.

Chris remembered running in the Tundra in his native home in Alaska and the freedom he felt of rolling down the hill—and not getting hit by any rocks, because there were no rocks. While recalling the memory, both Chris and I were struck by the parallel between the accident and his memory, the themes of spinning and not hitting. Let's see how this becomes meaningful in his process.

He spent one month in coma and then went through a long rehabilitative process that helped him regain most of his abilities. He describes his waking up as a psychedelic nightmare. All of a sudden he woke up in the hospital feeling totally disoriented and unable to remember anything that had happened.

When I started seeing Chris, his left side was weak and his balance was impaired. He was able to walk with one walking stick. He was acutely aware of the changes in his mind, such as his difficulty orienting himself in space, his problems with short-term memory, and his struggles pursuing the design work he loved so much and used to perform so easily. On the other hand, he finds himself confronted by his wife about changes in his temperament he doesn't grasp and he often remarks that what he expresses doesn't come out the right way. From his wife's and friends' reactions, he realizes that something is wrong. He remembers his old self and is learning to get to know his new self.

Chris is also feeling guilty as he sees how his process affects his wife and his child. Seeing the impact he has on his family, he starts feeling worthless because he can't provide for his family and help out as he used to, which leads him to become depressed and suicidal. He has enough awareness to notice that something is wrong, that what he wants to communicate doesn't come out right or comes out with more charged feelings than he is used to or wants to convey. These days his anger and frustration are more apparent and on the surface than they used to be, and he has difficulties controlling his feelings. His lack of emotional control strains his relationship and makes him feel depressed. He faces his limitations and recognizes that some of his emotions are "out of place," and he can't make sense of them. He describes his brain function as feeling like being in a fog, or playing a football game in the middle of a thick forest, or as a puppeteer who is not connected with the puppet.

When Chris had his accident his wife's life was traumatized, too. From one day to the next she was thrown into a new life. She had to cope with the fears of losing her husband, the challenges of becoming a caregiver, dealing with doctors and hospital staff, fighting for Chris's survival and the changes in her role as parent. With extreme courage and tenacity she stood by Chris's bed, talking to him and praying for his recovery. She organized his care and brought several healers to Chris's bedside to support his healing. Despite poor medical prognosis she never lost faith in Chris's ability to wake up from his coma. When I met her I was inspired by her positive energy and her sense of optimism. I experienced her as someone who can confront almost any challenge. For me she personified health and a fighting spirit. Chris, on the other side, was constantly reminded of his disability and impairments. The more she took on, the less empowered he felt. His negativity and depression scared and stressed his wife more than his actual physical and cognitive impairments. For her they were a turn off and led her to have difficulties being intimate with Chris, which then reinforced Chris's sense of worthlessness, a painful cycle for both of them.

Much of my work with Chris and his wife was about redefining health as we described in Chapter 3. In describing Chris's therapeutic process in detail, I would like to illustrate the various relationship levels: Chris's internalized relationship process between different parts of himself and his external relationship process with his wife. Individually, I helped Chris learn to see his process not only as a handicap but also as an opportunity for growth. One day I noticed him staring out of the window of my office. I asked him what he was experiencing while daydreaming and looking out of the window. He told me he was looking at the clouds and it reminded him of one of his favorite places to be, on the rooftop of his house. He said he just loved sitting on the roof and watching the sky. He said it reminded him of the vastness of the Alaskan Tundra. As a person with a brain injury, he experiences himself as being sloppy, unsteady on his feet, often losing his balance, and feeling almost drunk. He is "against" or bothered by that state and wants to be more sober and help out more. But when he is in touch with his dream-like state, and when, with my help, he follows the flow of his altered experience without any preconceived ideas, his experience of himself changes and he is able to re-connect with a sense of vastness and freedom. Spinning, rolling down, meditating, and letting himself feel altered allowed him to re-connect with a sense of being at home in his native Tundra and also more comfortable with his current state.

At a later session Chris told me that during his coma he had dreamt of a bear hunter and a fat man who tried to intervene and stop the bear hunter from killing the bear. The bear hunter aggravated the bear so that the bear finally ate the fat man. The dream reminded Chris of his grandfather who was a moose hunter in Alaska. I asked him about his association to the characters in the dream and he referred to the bear as representing "Fierce Order." And the fat man he felt was himself with his disability. I was struck by his unusual wording of fierce order. I was reminded of my own experience of Chris, of his powerful handshake, and of his problem controlling his anger in his relationship. Fierce made sense. Chris is intense; his whole process is intense. And somehow he associated some order to all of this. Together we interpreted the dream as the bear spirit wanting him to get back in touch with his ancestral nature—a driven fierce power and energy. Yes he was disabled, sick, and traumatized, and underneath all of that there was something else, too—a power that wanted to be met and reckoned with.

One big step in Chris's healing process happened when he traveled on his own back home to Alaska to visit with his father. In the relationship counseling I had helped Chris's wife to step back and disengage from the caregiver role. I had stressed the need for her to take care of herself and to ask for help from Chris and others. She needed to expand her experience of health to include being more "vulnerable" and recognizing the health in being less "competent." The circumstances had forced her into taking charge, which she had done in an admirable and inspiring way. For her own sake and for the sake of the relationship, I recommended that she step down from the role of a protector and let Chris discover his own physical, cognitive, and emotional boundaries. Seeing that Chris was making progress and discovering new ways to re-interpret his process and getting in touch with the bear spirit allowed her to step back and let Chris travel on his own. This in turn boosted Chris's confidence and helped alleviate his depression and hopelessness.

The last time I saw Chris he reported feeling better. He said his thoughts were getting more organized and he was now able to keep a thought or memory for about one week, which was much longer than before. He was discovering for himself the depth of his new experiences. For example, his hearing had become more sensitive since the accident and he was focusing on the little noises, the detailed clear and sharp sounds, and hearing everything. He was aspiring to become a story-teller, was drafting a book outline about his experience, and was working on developing some Internet tools for people with brain injuries.

The relationship dimensions in coma care are multiple. Chris, for example, had issues with himself. He was struggling with internalized memories of himself and his expectations of being a certain way. His existing self-image did not allow him to open up to his changed life experience. One way to interpret his process is in the context of internalized prejudice against a less "abled" body experience. Another relationship level was with his wife who wanted him to be more positive and had difficulties tolerating his depression. At a third level both Chris and his wife also suffered in relation to the attitudes of all of us who, as a culture and community, pathologize certain experiences and categorize heath in a very narrow way. Mainstream concepts of health don't include the diversity of experiences that come with processes such as aging, living with a disability or chronic disease, or going through the transitions and adjustments from a disease. By repressing and marginalizing all the symptoms that don't fit into our notion of health we marginalize our neighbors, co-workers, and partners who struggle with symptoms that are so strong that they don't have the privilege to ignore them any longer. As I helped Chris's wife to open up to her own disability and vulnerability, she was able to relate to Chris in a different way.

Gary described many of the relationship levels and processes that are relevant in Coma Work and drew attention to the fact that some accidents, heart attacks, and strokes may be preceded by relationship or emotional conflicts such as depression and suicidal tendencies. Families and other relationships are significantly disrupted by someone's coma process. As parents, partners, and caregivers, we are confronted with our own feelings and limitations. Suddenly we are pulled into a new role with new responsibilities while our regular life is going on as well. We have to take care of the family, our business, and our own needs for emotional support. Many caregivers feel they don't deserve to take care of themselves as long as their partner, child, brother, or sister is in a coma. They think they have it so much better in comparison to their loved ones. How can they even consider taking a break or enjoying life?

Furthermore, families and caregivers are also asked to make decisions and choices that are very difficult and challenge many family systems. End-of-life type questions such as the withdrawal of supportive measures might come up. Often conflicts arise about who will best speak for the person in coma? Who knows him or her best, and so knows what he or she would want? Who becomes the spokesperson and is allowed to represent or advocate for the person in coma? Advance directives are meant to ease these questions, but in my experience they often don't resolve the underlying relationship conflicts and family dynamics.

The "identified patient" disturbs the family system and the family becomes the client as well. Coma is both an individual and a collective process. Families and caregiver teams become polarized and *dreamed up*[3] to represent the various roles, positions, and beliefs that characterize the current cultural and community debate. Some individuals will stand for a feeling approach, others for a rational one; some will make a case for lucidity and awareness, while others want to make sure that their loved one is comfortable and not in pain. Because there is no unequivocal way to know what the comatose person feels or experiences, there is a lot of scope for interpretation and debate. This will often lead to conflicts. In my own experience most care teams opt for being very generous with doing whatever it takes to make the comatose person physically comfortable. Obviously this is very important. One problem, however, is that most pain medication also has an effect on consciousness. I witnessed many comatose persons who in an effort to "reach out" and be more active showed facial and body expressions that could also be interpreted as signs of discomfort. Using Process-oriented Coma Work techniques I always first try to support whatever activity or energy the person in coma is displaying before recommending palliation and pain medication. I try to put myself into the position of someone who wants to come out or is trying to express something and imagine how it might feel to be medicated.

Many family members don't have very much understanding about coma and brain injury. Some assume that either you are unconscious or you are conscious, and when you come out of a coma you do it quickly. It is like being asleep and being awake. However, this is not an accurate picture of how people recover from coma. Most people emerge from coma very gradually. Initial signs can be an eyelid that flutters, a small finger or hand movement, and later an eye opening but maybe still not registering any kind of recognition or tracking. Some of the initial signals can look like a grimace. People in comas have an altered ability to control their muscles. Movements come out in unexpected ways, which makes them difficult to interpret. There is a general notion that emotional expressions are universal and that certain body or facial signals are tightly connected with a certain feeling such as pain, anger, shame. etc.; however, with a brain injury that affects motor or muscle control and function, the circumstances are different. In our work we try to keep an attitude of curiosity and open-mindedness. Relating to the energetic quality of each signal appears to us to be more appropriate and helpful as it allows for more options and possibilities.

Besides a lack of understanding of coma that we all share, many feel helpless, too. Helplessness leads health professionals and family members to search for new treatment ideas. Some team members will want to be more active and perform various procedures; others will be more passive, wanting to hold off from intervening and wait to see how the natural course of the illness goes. Some will be more open to letting the comatose person die; others will want to fight for life and recovery. These dynamics need support and facilitation.

Many medical professionals and caregivers are absorbed with the body, its disease process and treatment, and they concentrate on analyzing a particular set of symptoms and solving problems associated with that set of symptoms. Few are interested in looking at a holistic picture of a human being and how this particular moment of disease or injury fits into his or her life story. This disinterest can certainly create tensions with family members. In addition, people who are comatose can't even ask questions on their own behalf. This will incite someone to step into the role of an advocate to speak on their behalf. Comatose people need advocacy for their cause. The fact that maybe 40 percent of people deemed to be in a vegetative state are in fact conscious means we need a change in attitude and more specialized treatment. On the other hand, some advocates can stir up conflict in a care team that will need facilitation help.

Sometimes family members become discouraged from spending too much time at their loved ones' bed side. This is often because many people don't know how to interact with someone who is not responsive or responds with unintelligible body signals. You can ease that problem by demonstrating simple interactive body work skills that can bridge this communication gap. At other times the opposite was true, and you have to encourage a wife, husband, partner, or parent to leave their loved ones with the experts and go home and get their own lives back on track. Some people need support to separate themselves from their loved ones as their process didn't include caring for a comatose person over a long period of time. Even though these actions are aimed at preventing burn out or supporting someone's individual process, they don't always come out well. I learned that first I had to help the individual to process their inner or outer conflict with a critical role that was there to advocate and fight for recovery or a role that was blaming them from abandoning their loved ones. Only after we had resolved this fight with the critical role were people able to move on.

Families have a different relationship and perception of their loved ones than professional helpers. Professionals sometimes think the family members are biased and not objective enough. Some family members will keep relating to the comatose person as if they were responsive and fully in possession of all their faculties. They keep relating to them in their everyday manner. On the other hand, family members may well spend many more hours at the bedside than the medical staff and will see or experience their loved ones' behavior in much more detail and with a different feeling attitude.

One family member said to me,

She is still alive, as I mentioned, and physically, she is in top shape . . . because she isn't talking it is hard to say how far "gone" she is as far as brain damage goes. She responds to us quite a lot—mimics our facial expressions like when I'm scrunching my nose, blowing a kiss, or she'll give a thumbs up and move her legs on command. These to me are all good signs, but they consider her to be in a light coma and unfortunately the doctors don't see as much response as we, her family, do. Maybe we are too hopeful and so we are seeing things that are just not real? Some days we get hardly any response and other days she follows us with her eyes and smiles at us.

This perfectly describes the frequent discrepancy between the professionals' perception of obtainable responses and what the family sees and experiences. Many family members don't understand why their loved ones are considered to be in a coma when they perceive so many signs that their loved one is responsive. For example, in one hospital where I worked we cared for Cenan, a 20-year-old Albanian man, who had suffered a severe brain injury from a car accident. Cenan stayed in our clinic for over three years. From a purely medical point of view he was in a continuous persistent vegetative state and we had not seen any response from him. His family always insisted that he was reacting to them and answering their yes and no questions with a hand motion, but the medical team did not believe them at first. It was only after I sat together with him *and* his family that I saw what we had missed before. When his family surrounded Cenan, he was clearly more awake and attentive. The communication style of the family differed strongly from that of the team of therapists in that they were mostly loud and emotional, while the therapists were more reserved and thoughtful. Only after integrating the new communication style into our therapeutic approach were we able to establish definitive communication and join Cenan in his world. Using the movement of his right arm over which he still had muscular control, he could indeed answer yes and no questions, which enabled us to help him regain control over some acts of care such as pain management and being moved when he was uncomfortable which he previously had to endure passively.

Cenan's case shows how complex and difficult the assessment of consciousness is. Our lack of experience and in Cenan's example, our inability to adapt to culturally diverse communication styles, influences how we behave and relate to people in seemingly nonresponsive conditions. The lack of diverse communication skills may also explain some reports of misdiagnosing persistent vegetative state in medical literature.[4]

Differences in perception and interpretation can lead to conflicts between professionals and family members. The professionals' expertise gives them a lot of rank and power, and families often have difficulties standing up for their experience and knowledge. Sometimes they will cave in and go along with the medical view or alternatively turn to outside sources of support to help strengthen their view. In many situations I have witnessed whole group processes and long discussions about the patient's state of awareness. In the United States this is further complicated because reimbursement of the cost of specialized rehabilitative treatments depends on the comatose person's responsiveness. There is often a lot at stake. Coma is never an isolated process; it affects nearly everything and everybody associated with the person in coma. It can strain a family to the point of collapsing, destroy the families' economic stability, jeopardize their future, and rearrange allegiances and friendships. Coma is a crisis for everybody involved. It also has a way of exposing our common humanness, fragility, and vulnerability, and determination to learn and grow from the crisis. It challenges all of us on an existential level.

Because the issues are so complex and existential, both family members and specialized health professionals need facilitation skills to navigate the ups and downs and the many issues that come up internally and interpersonally. Differentiating between practical, everyday issues, the emotional processes and the existential or spiritual questions can be helpful. Using a facilitative approach that allows all voices and viewpoints to be heard and validated can smooth the progress of finding consensus within the caregiving team. Because many of the issues are existential and highly emotionally charged, it can be helpful to assist all caregiving team members to meditate on and process their feelings, questions, and views about death and dying, their relationship process with the loved one, the grief and loss of the "old" self, and everybody's openness to discovering a new person. Introducing such a Process-oriented approach can reduce the communication barriers, relieve the pain and sense of isolation, and facilitate team discussions and decision making.

A skeptical voice in me comes up to balance my Process-oriented positivity. It says something like: "That is all good and well, but some people's processes with coma and brain injury are extremely dreadful, with unimaginable pain and suffering, with changes in personality, sense of self and the environment, psychotic symptoms, violence, etc. People end up institutionalized and sedated for lack of specialized care and also because no care makes a difference." To which I might respond, "Yes, that is true, too. There is much more research that is needed. Our approach is not the answer to all the open questions. Coma and the many remote and altered states of consciousness are processes that we don't understand well at all. Please join me in finding new avenues."

CONCLUSION

In the rehabilitation clinic in Basel, Switzerland where I worked, I had the opportunity to implement Process-oriented concepts and skills in the therapeutic program for brain injured patients. I worked individually with people in comas and taught the medical staff and friends and relatives of the patients some of the sensitive communication skills.

This approach had an unexpected beneficial effect on patients, family members, and professional helpers. Family members felt better supported in finding ways to relate to their loved ones. They felt less isolated and had a better chance of staying in a bonding relationship with their relatives through body and movement contact. The staff of nurses, doctors, physical therapists, and occupational and speech therapists reported feeling less burned out. They had to fight less against the heavy impairments of the comatose patient's state and were better able to develop a feeling for the patient's inner process and to interact with them. Communicating with the patient in a comatose state helps transcend the isolation of both patient and caregiver and enhances relationship, even with initially noncommunicative patients.

With our increased awareness of minimal signals and the patients' feedback, we were also able to improve our diagnostic abilities, discovering, for example, more patients who had *locked in* conditions (a situation where the patient is completely paralyzed while his cognition still functions), which we would have overlooked without these new communication techniques.

Chapter 5

The Spirit of Healing: Accessing the Healer in You and Your Client

As we redefine what healing is, we also need to reexamine who it is that is actually doing the healing. This chapter focuses on the inner healer present in all of us—patients and caregivers—and describes how to access this healer and bring it out. It covers the use of awareness and psychology to foster innate self-healing abilities. This takes us into the realm between psychology and spirituality in healing, and comes up particularly when we encounter or are involved in extraordinary, medically unexplainable cures that appear to be miraculous.

WHO IS THE HEALER?

Gary: Two different cases have challenged me to rethink my concept of what a physical body is and where the healers are—in the client, in myself, and in our work together. Growing up in a family with a very traditional medical perspective, I grew up thinking about my body in primarily physical terms: Gary, you have a sprained ankle, and this is how long it will take to heal. However, even as a small child I knew the body was more than physical. When I woke up sick with a fever, in the evening my mom used to tell me that if I still had a fever by the morning, I would have to go to the doctor. I couldn't stand going to the doctor because he always made me stay out of gym class and other physical activities for a ridiculous amount of time after being sick. So I used to go inside myself and visualize armies attacking the sickness in my body. In the morning my mom would put the thermometer in my mouth and that fever would have disappeared. At other times my pediatrician would tell me not to exercise with a fever or cold, so I would go home, lock my door and do calisthenics, and suddenly I'd be well again. I was always following something in addition to my physical body.

It wasn't until I was in my early thirties and met Dr. Arnold Mindell and learned about his concept of the Dreambody—the part of us that is much more than just our physical body, and includes our dreams, dreamlike experiences, and mythical natures—that I began to understand why what I did worked. Mindell's first book, *Dreambody*, introduces the concept of a body that is both physical and full of dreamlike expressions. As a young child, I had so many different kinds of warrior dreams about knights in armor, and I was always fantasizing about people with magical powers. When I accessed this dreamlike part of myself, my symptoms disappeared.

I also discovered something similar with my daughter. Particularly when she had fevers or stomach aches, I would push on her feet, and she would start kicking and punching and her symptoms would disappear on the spot. One day she hurt herself seriously by jumping on a couch and landing on her neck; I asked her to walk like someone with an even more hurt neck. She did, and started to walk in this funny way. I asked her what she was, and she said a bear, and that she remembered she had just dreamt about a ferocious bear that started dancing. I told her to try first playing like she was a ferocious bear and then a dancing bear. She did both of these, and instead of having to take her immediately to the doctor or hospital, as she was in so much pain, she started to run and play and said the pain was gone. I took this and many similar experiences into my work with my coma clients. Never the less, none of this prepared me for the kinds of cases I am about to tell you about, and yet my basic belief in the spirit in the body and its ability to heal never changed. I am convinced that our most powerful healer is deep within us.

To illustrate this I want to tell you about one of my most seriously injured clients who has given me permission to write about her over the years, but even so, I have changed her name and location to protect her identity. Tammy was in her thirties. She had had repeated marital troubles that became increasingly violent. One day, she left her comfortable home and went for a bike ride. Her husband drove after her and ran into her at full speed. As if this wasn't enough, he then got out of the car, beat her head in, and then picked up a piece of glass from the shattered car and slit her throat. Tammy's family called me in to see their daughter who lay dying in the hospital, on life support, having been given no chance of survival. I worked with her a few times and saw her potential to respond. I had the family bring in her son who wanted to see her, and Tammy was particularly responsive to him. I worked with her for a few days and saw increasing levels of responsiveness, but then I had to leave town and promised that I would return as soon as I could. The family was told that with the massive brain damage from her injuries, plus oxygen deprivation, Tammy would almost certainly die, and even if she lived, she would be a vegetable.

A short while after I left, the family called me to tell me that their daughter was screaming. I went back to work with her and found that despite the noises she was making she was still in coma. Her prognosis hadn't changed, even though she was much more present and alert. Then I noticed her fist clench and started to play with it. I thought this woman must have so much anger in her. At one point, she reached out to punch my hand; I was stunned, and then she began to repeatedly punch my hand. I saw that Tammy had pictures of whales in her room, so I assumed she liked whales. I told her she was a whale, way down under the ocean, and that she should remember to come up to the surface sometimes. I followed her as she went deeper under and then came close to the surface, and I told her she was a great whale. After doing this for about an hour, I left, and over the next day or so she came out of the coma.

The rest of the story is all about the many "she will nevers" that the family heard from the medical staff. First "she will never make it." Then, when she clearly was making it, "she will never be more than a vegetable." Followed by, "she will never move," then "she will move, but never stand even with a walker," and "she will stand but never walk," all the way to "she will walk but never without crutches." We were also told that Tammy would make noises but never words, then well maybe words, but not sentences; then maybe sentences, but never be understandable, etc. Later still we were told she can speak, but she will never think complex thoughts, or comprehend; and then when she confounded them on that one, too, we were told she would never be able to go back to school, and so it went on. Tammy's recovery was so unusual, and she caused so much cognitive dissonance that the staff didn't know what to do. I loved the staff, and they even invited me to staff meetings when I was in town to discuss her case, but she was so far out of the range of normality. It was as if a flying saucer had landed in the middle of the town and it was so unexplainable that people just ignored its existence.

After years of work, and with the help of many people, Tammy was eventually able to walk unassisted, speak perfectly normal, go back to school, finish her degree, and work out in a gym. She became so strong that no one had ever better mess with her again! And these are only the physical changes, but let's stop and discuss them first. How is this possible? Every time she was told she couldn't do something, Tammy became more determined than ever to do it, and she did. She was unstoppable. There she was, basically a murdered woman, defying all odds. She told me that she once ran into her neurologists in the hall of the hospital, as she was walking to her physical therapy sessions, and they literally stumbled they were so stunned to see her. She has something more than a physical body operating here. The following quote from Dr. Arnold Mindell's book the *Quantum Mind and Healing* might help us to understand who she has become. "The person emerging from a near-death experience always seems to me to be more human and conscious, capable of identifying with infinity and, at the same time, with the human species and all planetary life. This new person is on the path behind all paths. This path is likely behind all you do and have done, as well as all you dreamed you could have done."[1]

Tammy had become what I call a dream warrior. She was doing in this world things that seemed impossible from an ordinary reality standpoint. A dream warrior can accomplish tasks and heal themselves and others in ways that are beyond the realm of physical possibility. Her healing wasn't only for herself. Every time I worked with her, I came away with some renewed sense of energy and with a broader perspective. I told her she was like a spiritual teacher.

Tammy's personality was evolving also. She became clear and assertive in ways she had never felt before. She used to be a person who had trouble setting limits, and yet this new person, when tapping into her own unlimited energy, could set sharply defined limits with others. Someone who couldn't express anger easily became fluid with her anger. She was no longer afraid of anything or anyone. Career dreams became career realities. Fears of the required courses she would need to take became just the next challenge. She could look back on her previous life with a kind of critical detachment, understand how she had gotten where she ended up, and decide to change the whole basis of her relationship to men, to her children, and to her own and her ex-partner's family. Those of us who worked with her couldn't believe what we saw before our eyes. Steps in her healing which the physical therapists said would take years, Tammy would take in months.

My situation with Tammy was unique in that we worked together for about three years. I am convinced that part of her ability to heal physically was because she worked on the emotional levels at such depth. She managed to clear so many of her feelings with the man who attacked her that she was able to leave behind any sense of being a victim. She identified as a powerful woman who could use her power to do what she needed to do. She could literally feel left over feelings toward him, in certain muscles, inhibiting her walking, or in her throat inhibiting her speech, and we would work on helping her express her feelings verbally and in movement. She kicked, punched, and screamed her way to health, as well as having been much more analytic and understanding of where she came from and where she was going. We worked on her dreams as well, as they guided her from stage to stage. We worked through her transition from intensive care to rehabilitation at the hospital, to a nursing home, to a home for people with head injuries, to her own independent living apartment. If a new relationship possibility came into her life, we did a whole new level of emotional clearing of the past, and a new clarity about who she was and what she wanted in relationships came forward.

Almost inevitably Tammy also went through her low periods when the work was too intense, and the progress too slow, but she never gave up. She maintained her mothering connection to her children, and slowly she was able to spend more time with them again, and eventually they moved back in to her place. She has never stopped creating the life that she wanted for herself.

LESSONS LEARNED FROM WORKING WITH TAMMY

Who healed Tammy? First, she had a great team of doctors and nurses who saved her life. Then she had all kinds of wonderful physical therapists, massage therapists, occupational therapists, speech therapists, and other kinds of healers. And I also know that the Process Work I did played a central role in helping her to come out of the coma and to move through various stages of healing. Yet these same teams of healers have also worked with many other people, many with less serious physical problems than Tammy, and we certainly have not often witnessed a recovery where the person came back all the way and then some. All of these inputs were crucial to her recovery, but Tammy herself was the most important factor in deciding what would happen. When we say someone's name, we are usually referring mostly to their conscious personality. But whatever was present in Tammy that helped her come back was also present when she was in coma, in partial recovery, and at full recovery. I am going to call this Tammy's essence, or spirit. My answer to the question, who is the healer, is that all of us are healers together, but the greatest of all healers is the spirit of the person themself.

I am convinced that what comes through me when I work on someone in coma is also something deeply spiritual, which connects me with that deep, essential part of the other person. My spirit and Tammy's spirit danced a healing dance together.

I want to share with you a dream I had around the time I started working with Tammy. I dreamt that I had walked into a hospital ward, where people were lying in deep comas. I didn't know what I could do to help. Suddenly my hand became filled with energy, and I began pointing at different patients. I would point until the person would come out of coma, and then I would move on to the next patient.

Since that dream about four years ago, my Coma Work has changed and gone to a new depth. The Mindells have recently developed this whole approach of sentience, essence work, and Earth-based psychology,[2] which has deepened where I can go. I used to have to wait for those miracle moments to happen spontaneously, but now I can reach them through the specific steps of going down into the essence and being present there. What happens then is still up to nature and is miraculous, but by being present the chances are greatly increased. It is like fishing, if I go to the river with a pole and go to the right spot where the fish are, the chances are much greater than if I just put my pole in anywhere. For example, I still work with the arm muscles, with the eye movements, and with the throat to get speech activated, but more than ever now I let the spiritual come in. I often stop and meditate and gain guidance about what to do next. Sometimes I put my hands on the person and let this Knower in me guide my hands where to work. In Process Work we call the wisdom that flows through us *Process Mind*.[3] In my Aikido training we call this universal energy Ki. I have begun at times to put my hands near the point of injury and let healing energy flow. Of course, there are many healing and spiritual traditions that use the hands this way. Tammy was the turning point for me though, as she made me realize that if people are going to make this healing journey back from and through coma, there is something much bigger than any doctor, coma worker, or coma client that is at work, and we need to be able to connect with this for the healing to occur.

In much of this book we focus on not being attached to the role of the healer. By this I mean the traditional view of the healer as the one who fixes something or someone who is broken. For me the basic assumption behind this view is problematic, because I don't see people as broken, but as evolving and growing and developing. In the consensus view the healer moves in only one direction, toward restoring the full functioning of the coma person. Whereas what I am interested in is something different, the healing that happens through us that uses the practitioner as a channel for healing energy to pass through. This is hard to articulate with words, but once a practitioner experiences it, this feeling reality is easily recognized and understood.

I will try to describe what happens to me or through me when I experience this quality of healing. Often I become increasingly calm and increasingly energized. My hands seem to suddenly know where to go. The family may confirm that I am going from point to point where pain or problems or injuries have occurred. I often know things about the client's life and can guess things that the family agrees are correct. The client and I have connected and somehow information has entered another realm that is not just locally contained within that client's body. When I am doing hands-on work, I feel this special energy pouring through me, and the closest I can get to what is coming out of my hands is what I call love. I feel this incredible love for the person radiating through my hands. This is the healer, this love coming through me. In Chapter 7 on burnout, I refer to this as the *BIG YOU*,[4] the part that is both you and beyond you and that connects to something that is truly healing. It doesn't work if we identify with this in some kind of egoistic way. The more I do that, the more I seem to lose touch with the healing flow in the moment. The best explanation I ever heard of this was from a Native American, Grandfather Wallace Black Elk, who I was able to study with. He said that he himself can't heal anyone. However, he works with a spirit who comes through him who can do the healing. He described this spirit's ability to heal head injuries, and he demonstrated this work at a major medical research center.

Now all this doesn't mean that the ordinary Coma Work skills are not important. We must still train, know the form, and all the right words and touches to use to get connected with and facilitate the client's process. This healing energy coming through simply means that sometimes uncanny unexplainable things happen, where it feels like something beyond the coma worker's ordinary personality is working through them. Whenever I have seen miraculous healings occur, they have this quality of something beyond the ordinary sense of self.

This is not just a momentary experience I am describing. Certain clients have this kind of flow where everything falls into place, and they seem unstoppable. It is not just that they want to come back or their family wants them to come back, but what I call *IT*, something bigger behind the whole scene is behind their coming back, and all the right pieces just fall into place. I remember an acquaintance of mine who came out of coma after a heart attack. He lives far away from the nearest hospital, but the day of his heart attack he just happened to be right next to the hospital, and he just happened to have someone with him who did cardiopulmonary resuscitation (CPR). Even though they couldn't revive him, he just happened to come back, as if there were some guiding hand behind the whole thing. These days when I see him, I talk with him about what the universe might have in store for him, because at first he went into a depression following his extraordinary experiences, but now he is slowly finding his way again on his path.

Mindell describes this wisdom behind the universe and behind our individual lives in great detail in his book *Earth Based Psychology.*[5] I have learned how to do his exercises on sentient work and Earth-based work. So now I can put myself into a receptive state where this wisdom can guide me and move me. Yet I still sense something very mysterious and mystical behind all of this. I can wait for that guidance, but whether or not it comes is something like an act of grace.

The stories I have referred to here are all stories where people come back from coma, but in Process Work and in different indigenous traditions, there has always been a sense that healing can also mean releasing someone to move toward their death if that is their process. Process Work has Taoism as one of its theoretical roots, and in Taoism the masters are said to be so close to nature that their presence in a certain region could move weather fronts that were stuck. Using this model, the coma workers job then is two-fold. The first part is to know all about the signal work and verbal work that we train people in as part of the basic Process Work program. The second is to follow what we call the second training, which is more intuitive, shamanic work. So the Process-oriented coma worker can not only move the process through their hands-on, verbal, and family work, but can also move the process on through their own closeness to nature. The more we do this Earth-based essence work, the more this wisdom of the universe, this *Process Mind*, moves through us, and directs the work. We have seen this sometimes when certain coma workers walk into the room. Just their presence often gets a strong response from the person in coma. By opening to this direction, I am no longer polarized in favor of life and against death; rather I am open to following wherever nature leads us.

I am still personally a very hopeful person. I come from a Jewish background that is very dedicated both culturally and religiously to taking care of people and to keeping them alive. Yet sometimes it is just so clear to me that a person is done on this plane and ready to go. I would never push a person toward death, but I do hold that space and tell them they are free to follow themselves. I have also had a few clients who felt they weren't free to come back to life until I really supported them to also feel free to let go and die.

Several years ago a friend of mine was in a coma. My partner and I sat with his loved ones. We all felt he wanted to go, that he was finished on this plane. We did what we could with our Coma Work and saw his lack of response to almost everything we did. It was like he had already left, and just his physical body remained. We supported this going, as did his family, and about 10 days later, he died peacefully. His family asked us to bring our drums and to drum for him. He was Native American, and we sang and drummed and prayed for him in a large community gathering. We could feel his presence, both those of us who were mystics and the Catholic priest present at the service. I learned from him. He lived fully whatever he did, and he died the same way, with the same one pointed focus as he rode horses, built barns, and moved through life. Death was clearly just the next gateway for him. Again I bring this up not just to ease people's journey into death, but to show that when we polarize against death, we may actually freeze the process so that the person can't die and can't come back to life either. All of their energy is frozen in conflict. Working on the essence level we utilize our deepest selves and the power of nature to work with these conflicts so the river can flow again. We are the Taoists, the worshippers of the river, of flow, of freedom from polarization. This in itself is healing. Sometimes we call it death, sometimes life, but from this place of essence, it is just flow.

In conclusion, the Mindells say Process Work has a first and second training. The healer is the summation of all the first training, all the formal psychological and bodywork and medical and other information that comes through in our training and, additionally, they carry something special through them and have been through some kind of second training that opens them up to the spiritual, unknown, shamanic realms. Technicians can be highly skilled and a great support to the coma person and family, but the kind of healer I am referring to carries both these personal skills and something beyond the personal, they have the tools and take the time to go back to the wisdom that goes beyond their personal knowledge and personal resources. Healing is a combination of skills and our deepest connection to ourselves and the universe. For example, I may have highly trained hands, whether as a surgeon or bodyworker or coma worker, but if I am a healer, I am also in touch with the energy and guidance that come through my hands.

The first step in moving into these more sentient-based, shamanic healing powers is learning how to believe in them and access them. This exercise (Exercise 5.1) can help you learn to believe in yourself. Two of the most important pieces of this work are to tell the client to believe in what they are experiencing and for the coma worker to take the same

Exercise 5.1
The Power of the Open Healer (For Two People)

---

1. Connect with your own healing power. Feel the feelings that you have in your hands. Let yourself be open and see like a seer, around and into your client. Open up to your dreamlike information that is always in the background.
2. Let's experiment with the healing powers we have. Have your partner play like he or she is in a coma.
3. Feel your essence in your body. Notice where in your body you feel connected to the deepest part of yourself. Take a few minutes to center yourself through your connection to this essence. If you get stuck, feel this feeling in your body and associate it with a spot on the Earth that reminds you of this feeling. Go to that spot and let yourself become that Earth spot. Let it direct you.
4. Now imagine you have access to your deepest healing powers from this place of connection. Try working from this place of power.
5. Find out from this place what the person's process is, and rather than trying to heal him or her, watch the person's feedback, and help the person grow by being connected to your deepest self, so that he or she can connect with his or her deepest self.
6. Follow what happens from this place of deepest connection between you.
7. When you reach a place of momentary closure, gradually come back to your everyday selves and stay connected with your deepest self and stay connected to your partner. From this place of oneness with Self and other, ask the person for feedback about what he or she experienced.

---

medicine and learn to trust their own powers of healing. The purpose of this exercise is to learn more about these healing powers, and to allow them to flow through you.

Pierre: As a medical doctor I want to think that my knowledge, expertise, skills, interventions and prescriptions are what heal people, but I also know that people's behavior, for example, their compliance with my directions, is relevant to the outcomes. It is significant then, that in the United States more than 30 percent of doctor's prescriptions are not followed and yet some people get well anyhow. Others who do follow their doctor's prescriptions *and* live a healthy lifestyle may nevertheless become or remain sick.

Obviously, modern medicine has made much progress, and many of us are now able to live longer, healthier lives because of the progress made. However, I also know that my clients' psychology and their emotional intelligence have a significant influence on their health and ability to heal. Social circumstances such as education, money, and other resources also have a strong impact on health and people's ability to stay healthy and heal. What is health and what promotes or hinders healing is complex; many intertwined factors contribute to the outcome. Health itself is a difficult and complex concept with probably as many definitions as there are people in this world and in healing there are many intangible factors that elude us.

Personally, I have found Arnold Mindell's description of the three levels of experience[6] helpful to give me some orientation. On a consensus reality level, our health is determined by mechanistic determinants, for example, the level of the health professionals' hard skills and knowledge, the clients' behaviors, and the social dynamics. On the dreaming level there are psycho-emotional as well as relational processes that determine the course of a disease process. And on a sentient level you are spiritually whole, no matter what, sick or well.

Let me give you an example from my own experience. About four years after immigrating to the United States, I became sick. I was having diffuse abdominal pains that came and went without a recognizable pattern. I was under considerable stress finishing my dissertation for my PhD, working as an underpaid mental health counselor, and going through the difficult process of applying for permanent residency in the United States. I treated myself for possible stomach ulcers without much success. One night the pains were so strong that I had to go to the emergency department. There, the doctors quickly diagnosed me with having gall stones and an inflamed gall bladder. They recommended immediate surgery, which they performed very well. But after the surgery my blood markers didn't return to normal levels. Through the intermediary of nurses, doctors recommended a second surgical intervention to release some blockage they assumed was remaining. The surgeon didn't have time to come and explain the situation to me in person. I remember lying in bed and, because of my own training, knowing a lot about the medical process, but feeling anxious and getting more and more frustrated about the lack of communication between my doctors and me. I then remembered my dream of the night before. I had dreamt of a big cathedral that had a small chimney that was blowing off steam under a lot of pressure. A friend helped me over the phone to work on that dream and got me in contact with my own anger about the lack of appropriate communication. I also got in touch with my own core beliefs and values and felt re-empowered.

Later that evening, a nurse told me that the doctors had decided to check my blood again before making a final decision about surgery. I had to remain without eating to be ready for surgery. In the middle of the night my IV got blocked and had to be exchanged. In my own mind

I still felt hopeful about my chances of not having to have the second surgical procedure done, and so I asked if they could wait before giving me another IV. The poor nurse had to go back and forth communicating with me and the doctor on night duty. I got so fed up that I asked that the doctor come in person to explain his reasoning and what he wanted me to do or agree to. I told the nurse I wouldn't have her do anything to me before I was able to talk to the doctor myself. The poor resident on night duty had to pay for the lack of overall communication between the doctors and me, but after another hour he came and we had a good chat and I agreed to get another IV, despite the fact that I thought it might not be necessary. The most intriguing part of that process was that after all that emotional processing, my body reacted by letting go of built up fluids and internal pressure. In the morning they took my blood and everything was back to normal, and I was able to be discharged the same morning without further surgery.

What healed me here and prevented the second surgery? How was my anger and frustration connected to the temporary blockage? How was my insistence on fair treatment and communication related to me letting go of the buildup of water in my body? Did the reduction in interstitial fluids reduce some swelling that had been contributing to the blockage? I also remember that on the phone I had been able to process deep feelings about my current experience in the United States. The U.S. laws and regulations hadn't accepted my Swiss medical training and didn't allow me to practice as a medical doctor, which humiliated me. As an alternative to going back to medical school, I had chosen to do a second training in health psychology. This had forced me to start at the bottom again. The lack of communication with the doctors had reinforced my sense of not being recognized and respected as a colleague. I was feeling low not only because of being sick but also about my experience of not being validated for my medical knowledge and experience.

This whole process taught me that there are many factors that contribute to healing which go beyond hard medical skills and technical interventions. In my case the surgery was necessary and professionally executed. But then my healing was also embedded in a relevant personal psychological and emotional context. Both medicine and psychology have a lot to add to healing. In my view, psychology allows us to access the body's innate healing powers. Facilitating the body's dreaming process and the emotional dynamics between the parties involved in the healing process are powerful tools that complement and enhance the effectiveness of medical interventions.

These cases and personal stories show that the healer is a combination of consensus reality medical interventions, alternative medical interventions, the individual's awareness process, and the way nature moves this process. Part of what is so fascinating about Coma Work is that we are often working where consensus reality interventions have come to their limit, where nothing else can be done that isn't being done. This place of limit is for us just the beginning of exploring what is possible beyond consensus reality interventions.

We have been focusing on the healer within ourselves as clients and as coma workers. In the next chapter, we explore how we can utilize our own altered states in our work with our clients.

Chapter 6

Using Your Own Altered States to Benefit the Person in Coma

When we work with coma patients, it alters our own states of consciousness as practitioners and family members and we need to know how to make these states useful. This chapter helps us get comfortable with our own altered states and learn how to access them, and what to do when we find ourselves pulled into our own altered states by the depth of the coma person's experience. Exercises are included that focus on learning how to ride the wave of your own altered states.

Pierre: In previous chapters we explored definitions and concepts of health and healing and the forces behind individual healing. The experience of illness has many facets. It is comprised of the subjective experience of the symptoms, the emotional states that accompany the symptoms and is influenced by the relationships that surround us and our symptoms, and the many social aspects that the illness is embedded in. Another aspect of experiencing illness, and specifically of coma, is altered states. Altered states, or nonordinary states of consciousness, range from the mild dreamy or foggy states that accompany fever or fatigue to deep comatose states. They can include dreamlike visual and auditory experiences of a changed reality. These often go beyond what we usually include in our sense of what is normal and acceptable and they change our perception and experience of our bodies and the world around us. Altered states can be induced by mind-altering processes such as injuries or degenerative brain processes; psychiatric disorders;

substances such as alcohol, marijuana, and other drugs; holotropic breathing or hyperventilation; spiritual or cultural trances; meditation; hypnosis; peak experiences from extreme sports, sex, and music, etc. They are part of everybody's experiences, often pursued within specific subcultures or social contexts, but because of their inherent nature of breaking the boundaries of everyday reality they can also create anxiety and insecurity.

In ancient medicine or so-called primitive medical practices, altered states were and are used to access knowledge from other dimensions, worlds, and spirits. In many cultures shamans deliberately alter their consciousness to obtain knowledge and power for healing from the "spirit world." Other traditional healers use practices and rituals to induce altered states, which are considered conducive to healing. Spiritual healers use prayer, laying on of hands, music, and other rituals for individual and collective healing purposes. In Western scientific medicine, mind-altering substances are currently used in treatment of chronic pain (for example, medical marijuana), to assist psychotherapy, and sometimes in end stages of cancer to relieve anxiety. Alternative or complementary medical practices use progressive muscle relaxation, biofeedback, hypnosis, imagery, and meditation as techniques for accessing altered states of consciousness in which certain forms of healing can occur.

Nevertheless, the social controversy about the use or benefit of altered states is very polarized and elicits strong emotional reactions on all sides. It infringes on people's core beliefs about life and the meaning of it. Some subcultures oppose any form of losing control or fear the powers of altered states. And some individuals have a propensity for extreme states and need more grounding.

Process-oriented Coma Work is open to exploring what people experience: their fears and insecurities, their need for grounding, as well as their altered states of consciousness. It acknowledges the fact that many people go through stages in their disease process that come with changes in their ordinary states of consciousness and that these states can be meaningful. However, not everybody is as open. Many caregivers and medical professionals react with skepticism and mistrust when confronted with the idea of exploring altered states. The idea of integrating altered states as a source of wisdom that can benefit the healing process may be a challenging concept. For example, in mainstream medicine, many expressions of altered consciousness such as agitation and excitement tend to be quickly medicated and calmed down. Most health care professionals perceive these states as uncomfortable or distressing and will prescribe medication to ease the distress. I do believe that bodily comfort and minimizing distress is important, but I also think that careful listening to the dreamlike fantasies in delirious and confused states brings insights and opportunities for healing and personal growth, and it can lead to more sustainable comfort and overall well-being.

To introduce an approach that is curious about altered states requires tact and negotiation. It is useful to understand your own discomfort and apprehensions so that you can relate to other people in the care team. If you marginalize the deep-seated fears and polarized dynamics around altered states and their value and use, you might encounter resistance and skepticism. For many caregivers the priority is about practical issues such as regaining and maintaining skills and functions and relieving pain and distress. Process-oriented Coma Work introduces new approaches of treating people as they go through transitional altered states of consciousness. These methods can be perceived as a threat to the usual ways care teams and family members take care of their loved ones and patients. The outcome of every multidisciplinary effort depends on each team member's ability to work together and appreciate the value of the team's diversity. Facilitating differences of opinions and being open to learn from others are prerequisites for good teamwork and positive outcomes.

THE ALTERED STATES OF THE PRACTITIONER: JOINING WITH THE COMA PERSON

Gary: I want to expand here on what Pierre has begun to address around altered states and comas by bringing in some of my personal experience. Working with coma patients has always put me in altered states of consciousness. When I first began, I would have to go for a walk to ground myself after working on someone before I could drive because I was too much in the other worlds. Now I have learned to go into and out of those altered states more consciously. I continue to have my own mystical experiences and try to bring these in to my work with the clients. First, I drop into my own center and connect with my own essential nature. Since beginning my psychological work with people, I have always had moments where I suddenly know something about someone; however, the psychic connection I feel and make with people in comas is at a whole different level. With the person in coma, all kinds of connections occur as I narrow that gap and discover the common worlds between my client and me. Dr. Amy Mindell puts it this way in *Coma, a Healing Journey* when she says, "Even if you do not have many skills, a comatose person responds well to the loving attention with which you try to join in and adapt your communication style to the altered state of the comatose person."[1] Somehow the client's altered state gives me permission to go with the person into altered states more than if my client is in a place of more consensus reality. My hands work differently, as I let them go where they are guided to go. Often family members will comment how I went right to an injured spot, or right to where the physical therapist or other therapist had been working. Next, I get information about the person's life that I can often have confirmed by family members. It might be something about their childhood or any current or past part of their life, or information about their health issues. I will often get information that I believe is about what their journey is like in their coma, or what might be stopping them from coming back further into a conscious state.

Before I started to include sentient work in my Coma Work, I used to stay close to the sensory-grounded material, but now I often leap into the sentient realm. Sensory grounded relates to what I can see, hear, touch, and access and experience through my senses, and sentient sparks off this, but then goes into my deepest feeling and my clients' deepest feeling, We are in the realm of being pre-verbal, that is, those moments before we can speak of our experiences. These kinds of experiences depend not on noticing signals but on catching flirts. Flirts are a kind of flicker awareness at the outer limits of our perceptions. We may not be able to pin a flirt down to a signal because it is gone almost as soon as it arises.

One of the clearest cases of this use of both signals and flirts was when I was working on a man who had been in a plane crash. Despite the medical prognosis that he had no chance of any kind of recovery, I felt this man's presence from the moment I walked into his room. Much of my work with him was following sensory-grounded work. I went from channel to channel, working with the responsiveness in his lips and the movements in his mouth. I stimulated these parts of him, and placed my hands on all the different parts of his body involved in speaking. I also appreciated the movements he was making with one hand, and worked with his fingers to help him increasingly reach out more and more with his arm, hand, and fingers. I also worked with relationship, particularly on how close he would get to his wife and his son, and respond with his eyes and by moving his neck toward the people he was closest to in life. I was also interested in how much movement he had in one side of his body, and none on the other, and so I worked with following and amplifying even the most minimal nano-movements on the inactive side, and helped him develop much more movement in this side. I worked with his physical body and with his emotions as I saw them arising.

I also asked him all kinds of yes and no questions, getting him to move his arm for yes and to stay still for no. The most important answer I received was that he was interested in coming out of this coma and wanted to come out in about a month. He gave the strongest feedback when I asked what kinds of things would be the most powerful draws to help him come back to consciousness, and he said it was his feelings of family and his work to help other people. He gave little feedback to returning to his job. This is usually as far as I might have gone, although I might have made some preliminary guesses into what this coma state was about for him.

However, with sentient work, I could go much further. Something he did caught my attention. In sentient work we call this catching a flirt. His eyes moved back for just a brief moment and he looked at the light, and he had a look on his face that seemed to me like something ecstatic. I let myself go there with him, and suddenly I felt like I was in the realm of angels. It was such a beautiful experience, and it went on and on. I actually have this on a videotape. When I came out of this ecstatic state, I did something I have never done before. I gave his wife a specific prediction that he would come out in about three weeks and begin speaking. In about three and a half weeks, I got a call from her saying that he was speaking, but could only speak about God! I understood completely because of what we had gone through together. I knew he had been very active in the church before his coma, but his wife said he had never talked about God nonstop in this way. Going into this sentient work allowed me to be present in that place where I think miracles occur.

Months later I began to dream about similar protective spirits that were there for me. Was this his work, my work, or both of ours together? I think that this was a shared space we were both heading toward, and that we went so deep together we entered into a shared world. It was a different world, one that the quantum physicists would call a parallel world, to consensus reality. My going into this world with him, when in coma, allowed me to communicate with him about God, about his oneness with God, and about being a vehicle for bringing that God energy back into this world. In Process Work, we talk about the spiritual channel as one of the main channels of experience. Yet, until my work with this man, I hadn't quite known how to build this in, how to catch a flirt like this and go deeply into some kind of shared essence place. With this man I had the courage to talk about his coming back soon because of the power of what I experienced with him.

These parallel worlds are always accessible, but Arnold Mindell has often said that it takes some kind of life crisis to take us to these places.

He had his angelic state, and I had a similar kind of angelic-like experience the last time I had a huge life crisis; I was caught in a very stressful work situation that I felt I couldn't get out of. Then suddenly, just as I was getting out of it, I lost a huge amount of money and felt I couldn't leave until I turned things around. I was tired, sleep-deprived, stressed, and unhappy. My moods were affecting my work, relationships, and other parts of my life that mattered so much more to me than this troubled financial scene. Then I had a dream of this incredible presence who told me that they were always right there with me, and I calmed down. Within a month or so, the situation turned around, and I was able to free myself.

One of my friends, let's call her Frieda, told me the following story that her mom told her; even though her mom wasn't in a coma, she had a very similar angelic-like encounter. Her mother was in the middle of chemotherapy for cancer and was terrified because she had been given a new chemotherapy drug that the doctor told her might make her more ill. Frieda had given her a tape of spiritual kinds of music. Her mother wasn't someone who had mystical experiences and would have described herself as a mainstream person. However, she told me of the following experience during one of her sessions. She was holding her husband's hand and focusing on the music, and then she saw her dead aunt holding her right hand, her grandmother her left hand, her father was holding her head, and there were six angels standing all around her. The angels started swooping from toe to head and kept circling her with light for an hour and a half, filling her with light. There was so much love present that she couldn't speak, and she put her head under the covers to hold onto the state and cried during the whole treatment. She peaked over the covers and looked into the room where everyone was getting chemotherapy and all the people had angels around them, and all the nurses had angels following them, with the angels hands on the nurses back sending light into them. She couldn't talk about the experience for about 24 hours, and burst into tears when she told her husband and daughter. She knew she was healed and that she would make it through the chemotherapy with positive results, which is exactly what happened. Now this wasn't a coma, but I am convinced that these are the kind of states that coma patients go into. This is why I often tell family members to be careful how they interpret the expressions the coma patients have on their faces. They may not be just ordinary expressions of pain and pleasure, but expressions of worlds that many of us know only in our deepest dream states and deepest states in the middle of the night.

Many indigenous cultures know it takes these extreme moments to connect with these essence places. In part of my training I spent many hours with Native American elders in sweat lodges. After many hours of heat, the worlds began to open up and alter. I would suddenly feel myself in connection with the trees, or with different animals, or with people far away. Yet, we have become so far away from these experiences that perhaps the chemotherapy and coma wards are like the sweat lodges and other similar practices such as sun dances, where people can connect with the forces of the Earth and the spiritual realms.

This Earth-based work that we have learned in Process Work has always been a part of nature. When I first began my therapy practice, I was living out in the country and wanted to raise goats. I went to buy goats from this very pleasant woman, and when she found out I was a therapist, she asked me if she could tell me something that she hadn't ever told anyone. She said that she had had a terribly hard childhood where she never really had a mother. One day, when out in the garden, she suddenly began to cry and cry, and she threw herself on the ground. She suddenly felt this warmth radiating from the Earth, which enveloped her in the most beautiful loving light she had ever experienced. She heard the words in her ears that the Earth was her mother, and she was not alone, and after this her life changed. She no longer felt like a woman who had always psychologically been an orphan. In coma, we also meet these kinds of Earth-based experiences that our ordinary consciousness doesn't usually allow.

I have never had a client yet who didn't say that they came out of coma transformed. What is it that brings about this transformation? I am convinced that it is these kinds of spiritual experiences that the person has while in the comatose state. I am aware of one person in Arizona who is researching these states by hypnotizing people after they come out of coma and studying what they say they experienced while in coma. It is too early to speak in detail about what he is finding, but he indicated to me that people were aware of everything that went on in the hospital room; could remember things that were said, which he had been able to verify with other family members who were present, and were having these other-world ecstatic experiences.

Is it possible that people in comas have access to both of these worlds simultaneously but can't communicate about either of them? Maybe when we are not in altered states, we can communicate but not go as deeply into these worlds simultaneously. I have always felt that part of my job as a coma worker was to help build these bridges between the world of coma and the world of the waking, between the nonordinary world and the everyday world.

There is generally something in the more mainstream attitude that says, "Get out of that coma." I saw it so clearly when one of the clients

I was working with would grab his son and tell him to get out of that coma and come and help him at work. I totally understand the feeling, and would feel the same way as a parent. However, as a coma worker, my job is to facilitate between these states. If the son could talk, he might say something like, "Dad, I would like to come out but I am busy in here. I am not even sure what I am doing in here, but it is very different from your world." In my role as facilitator, I often say to both sides something about changing. I might say to the son that if he comes out I will help him stay in contact with and live out some of the states he has found and experienced. I might also say to the father that he might want to spend time exploring other parts of his life besides his working 70 hours a week. Maybe they will meet somewhere in a different kind of world besides work. Maybe they will meet in the father's world, maybe in the son's world, and maybe in some new place that is both of their worlds.

In Process Work, we have always had this concept of negotiating and moving between these two states, but mostly we apply this approach when working with extreme psychiatric states. What this basically means is that I don't just value either the psychiatric or the mainstream state, but facilitate between the two. Thus, if a person is in an extremely manic state, I might interact with him from a more ordinary state of consciousness, and then also take his side where he is currently in mania and mediate between the two states. The idea is that if I just polarize against this state, I might lock him into it more, and if I just support this state I might cut him off from integrating it with the more mainstream state. I take a similar position in Coma Work. If I just go against the state, I might unintentionally prolong it. This is one of the reasons why we always tell people in comas to believe in their experiences. The general idea is that the more you believe in what is happening and the deeper you go into it, the shorter the period you spend in the extreme state. However, if I over-glorify this coma state, partially as a compensation for a more mainstream model that views this state only as pathological, then I may also cut the person off from becoming more fluid with the outer mainstream world and from being able to move in and out of their altered states.

The best example I have of successful work like this goes back to Herman who was unemotional before the coma, came out of the coma by being very feeling and following his feelings, and then integrated these feeling states into his relationships with his family before he finally died. He may very well have needed the coma to go so deeply into his emotions, but then the real point was to come out and use all of this new emotional power in his relationships. So I encouraged both going deeply into himself, and then coming out and being with his family. These are not just personal or family issues, but also collective issues. We live in a culture where it is extremely hard to maintain our balance and, for example, be very successful in the world and to be really present for our families and take care of our bodies and other parts of our lives. For him, the coma in some ways allowed him to find this balance between his business and his emotional worlds.

Is it possible that a person would unconsciously seek out or stay in these states to be able to have these experiences? Maybe we will go to incredible extremes to reach these states because they are more vital to us than almost anything but life itself. Is it possible that hanging on the precipice between life and death may be a necessary place to meet these forces that can reconnect us to the meaning and purpose of life? Why do some people come back and some die and some stay in the exact same place in coma? These are some of the central questions that remain for me. However, I don't expect answers to all of these questions, because coma allows us to stare into the mystery and wonder and dream and question, and this is in itself so important. All of these questions also suggest research projects, for example: Are there fewer comas in indigenous cultures that regularly take people into deep altered states as part of ritual? Do people from cultures where people are trained to go in and out of altered states who do go into comas spend less time in them?

PREVENTION OF COMAS

I have just suggested that maybe one way that people enter into an altered state of consciousness is by going into coma. I also mentioned that in indigenous cultures there are often rituals that connect people with these states. In Process-oriented Psychology, we utilize sentient methods to go into these realms. Many of the drug addicts I have worked with have described their addictions as failed attempts to connect with these deepest parts of themselves. If my theory is correct, then the more we are able to pick up these deepest states, the less likely we are to go into coma.

Depression may also be a sign of this lack of contact with this essential nature and it is common knowledge among coma workers that almost all of the people we have worked with have a history of depression, or have had some kind of significant depression within the previous year. Although this isn't universally true, as I have worked with a few people whose partners were sure that they weren't depressed, even so working on depression in one's life may help prevent coma. When we lose contact with this deepest part of life, we become anxious and depressed. Also, certain kinds of depression take us down deep into ourselves, and if we go far enough down and don't fight this type of depression, it actually leads us into feeling connected with the Earth and the deepest levels of our own experience. The challenge is to find a way to connect with these deep states without the hardship that coma brings. Part of the work of personal development is to learn to move fluidly between our ordinary states of consciousness and daily life and our altered states of consciousness.

One of the most interesting pieces of research I do with my students is to ask if anyone has ever been in a coma. If they have I then ask them if they have had repeated experiences where they knock themselves out or come close to this. Several have said yes, which implies to me that these altered states tend to repeat themselves, which gives weight to the idea that they are meaningful and trying to put the person in contact with certain core experiences.

Thus, the more we consciously take time to go into our altered states and explore them; the less likely it seems that we will need to go into comas. This also suggests the collective nature of these states, for example in societies such as the United States that never stop, that are totally extroverted, then coma looks like the most extreme representation of what *isn't* happening in that society. In a very extroverted, Western culture, it is hard to find enough time and space to go inside and be quiet and meditate for a few minutes, and it can become very difficult to live out this kind of deep internal state on a regular basis. Try going into a crowded shopping mall and then into a coma ward. It is quite remarkable that the two can exist in the same city, and yet maybe they are related to each other, as the extreme internal, nonmaterial state, that is the closest state to death without being dead, is some kind of balance to the materialistic externally driven lives we lead.

Dr. Amy Mindell says something similar in her book *Coma, a Healing Journey*:

Coma work awakens all of us to the often unnoticed depths of human experience. It brings each of us to the brink of the most elemental questions about life, about death, and about the meaning of human existence. Perhaps contact with comatose people will remind us of the vastness of our own experience and will propel us to draw us closer to the profound inner stream that guides our lives. As we enter this current state, we live more fully, throughout the eternity of life.[2]

SOME CENTRAL LIFE QUESTIONS THAT COMA WORK RAISES

After having now examined the approaches I take to Coma Work, I want to focus on some of the central questions this work raises. These aren't meant to be answered, but to be pondered, explored, and researched. I have mentioned several of these throughout the book, but here are a few:

- Why do some people go into coma and come out and others do not?
- Why do some people take coma as a path of awakening whereas others take different paths?
- If someone could die rather than be in a coma, why would they hang on?
- How does the brain repair what appears on CAT scans and fMRIs to be irreversible damage?
- How do comas positively transform individuals who come out?
- How do they transform families whether or not the person comes out?
- What do our needs for contact, sexuality, and other forms of intimacy have to do with coma?
- How effective are spiritually based methods with coma patients?
- Do they work equally well with someone with a previous connection to spirituality and someone who didn't have this connection before coma?
- How far are comas preventable?
- How accurate are loved one's dreams about the person in coma and about the future of that person in coma?

These are just a few of the hundreds of questions I hope will be researched in coming years. In the last chapter, Pierre and I begin to address some of these questions more directly.

Chapter 7

Preventing Burnout

Family members and caregivers who provide care for coma patients, long term and in difficult circumstances, can develop symptoms of burnout. This chapter helps family members and caregivers to utilize their own sense of fatigue and hopelessness to guide them to their deeper healing powers. The methods we describe will help transform stress into "vitamins" for sustained healing and will help caregivers avoid becoming stuck in the role of constant caregiving in which they focus so much on the patient that they tend to marginalize their own needs and processes. This chapter explains how to remedy this imbalance.

Pierre: Burnout is a set of experiences that includes emotional exhaustion, fatigue, distress, feeling numb and lacking care, feeling overwhelmed, out of control and unproductive, and much more. It is associated with depression, alcoholism, drug abuse, and suicide. It occurs most frequently among professional people in the helping or caring professions such as teachers, nurses, social workers, counselors, and doctors. Family members and other caregivers of people with serious illness or disabilities may also have similar experiences of burnout.

The process of burnout has many facets, including intrapersonal, interpersonal, and systemic factors. Internalized pressures and expectations, such as wanting to be a good doctor, mother, and partner; our personal coping resources, or lack thereof, also influence our chances of developing symptoms of burnout. Relationship factors are also relevant such as the individual and cultural expectations and our desire for doctors who meet our expectations of being experts who don't show their uncertainty or vulnerability. The way we behave as "victims" when we are sick and defer to our helpers while, at the same time, feeling jealous of the privileges they have can also have a significant impact. Many doctors and other helpers feel personally criticized for systemic or structural failures and limitations and feel they can't fight back because of the privileges they have. I remember working in Senegal and learning that, among the local community, jealousy was thought to be one of the main factors causing illness. The experience of rank, power, and privilege, of being the helper and not the helped comes with a double bind—your own needs become marginal and irrelevant. The role of the sick one can make others sick, too. Obviously, we experience situations in which we are helpless and in need of someone taking charge, and the feeling of being a trusted helper is also empowering. On the other hand, if that role isn't shared and fluid, if the helper one-sidedly identifies with the role of helping and marginalizes both their own need for help and the power of the person they are helping, it will eat him or her up. Equally, if as "victims" we marginalize our own power to help and other people's need for care, then we co-create both our own helplessness and the burnout in our helpers.

Burnout also has its roots in systemic dynamics and failures. It is a symptom of a diseased health care system in which most of the resources are spent on treating narrowly defined illnesses caused by infectious, genetic, and metabolic agents and other processes that can be fixed by operative and other mechanical procedures. Most knowledge, training, time, and money are focused on acute situations that require a high level of expertise and control from the medical system. Unfortunately over 70 percent of patient care doesn't fall into this category of high acuity requiring specialized expertise. Most care evolves in a chronic, complex, and messy environment in which control remains strongly in the hand of the chronically ill person, his or her family, friends, co-workers, and spiritual mentors. Chronic diseases are the leading cause of death and disability in the United States.[1] In chronic care management clients have primary control over decisions and learn to live with their symptoms. As helpers our job is to accompany our clients and their families on their individual journeys of healing and transformation and support them to live a meaningful life despite or with their symptoms.

Most illness experiences and processes are also influenced by our beliefs and values and by social dynamics such as financial status and education, racism, sexism, and homophobia, which are not under the control of either the helper or the patient. The current doctor-/expert-centric medical model is failing both the patients and their helpers. Most patients need more than acute medical care. They need housing, jobs, and adequate insurance. Most doctors and other helpers are not trained to navigate the messy and complex demands that their patients and clients bring with them that do not respond to quick fixes and prescriptions. The helplessness that we face vis-à-vis emotional, relational, and social challenges often overwhelms our ability to cope. Other administrative and systemic pressures such as heightened accountability and responsibility, as well as increased bureaucracy, mean the whole system is getting very sick and is on the brink of collapsing.

As caregivers of a comatose and/or a severely injured and disabled person, we are facing enormous challenges. Especially as a family member or partner you are suddenly thrown into an abyss of extra work, financial difficulties, loss, and grief. As the "survivor" you almost automatically react by pushing all of your own needs aside. You are there to help your loved one who is going through this extremely difficult experience. Nobody will even consider whether being a caregiver was part of your plan, or if it fits into your views of how your life was going to unfold in the future. Everybody and especially you will expect yourself to shape up to the challenge and do what it takes to ease whatever is happening to your loved one. In the balance of who needs support, who is suffering, helpless, and in pain, the needs of the person in coma will always outweigh your own. Self-care doesn't exist in the caregiver's mind. It has no place given what our loved ones are going through. Taking a break may be accompanied with enormous guilt and at times can be emotionally and psychologically impossible. The lack of accessible specialized care makes it even more difficult, because we often have to leave our loved ones behind in a worse than deplorable care environment.

In my experience partners and families become very resilient. They develop extra energy, bring people together, and become community and social activists for the cause of their loved ones. On the other hand, burnout is almost inevitable. The strain is so extreme that it is often only a matter of time until the stress takes its toll. It sometimes manifests itself in conflicts within caregiver teams; it comes up as feelings of resentment toward the loved one and also in caregivers becoming sick themselves.

On an individual level, relieving burnout requires stress management and other coping skills such as mindfulness, relaxation, and meditation. It also involves the development of relationship skills and both social and systemic change. Stress is a subjective experience and what is experienced as distress varies from one individual to the other. Personal values, expectations, ethics, and morals, personal upbringing and life experiences such as trauma and/or privileges all contribute to individual resilience and coping mechanisms. In my own research I have found that our individual subjective experience of empowerment based on psychological, spiritual, and social factors has a significant impact on our ability to handle life challenges and stay well. Antonovsky[2] and other researchers have shown that our ability to see our life course in a meaningful and manageable manner is strongly related to positive long-term health outcomes.

Process Work has developed soft and hard skills to improve meaning at both individual and community levels. These skills can be used to combat burnout from a personal and systemic perspective. Process Work takes a homeopathic approach as we believe that the solution to the problem lies within its symptoms. Fighting against burnout or simply soldiering on will often make symptoms worse. Following the nature of the experience is the key to finding meaning and overcoming burnout. We recommend helpers to reconnect with their original vision that motivated them to engage in the path of helping. Idealistic, altruistic individuals are drawn to the helping professions because it is a wonderful, challenging, and incredibly humane endeavor. Facing our limitations and inadequacies brings us to our growing edges. The burnout symptoms force us to slow down and re-evaluate our own path and direction as well as the manner in which we follow our path. For some it might resolve in a change of direction and career. Others may need to reconnect with their own inner strength and motivation. A good way to get in touch with our source of wisdom and power is to follow the experience moment by moment. Exercise 7.1 helps us explore the individual meaning of our own burnout experiences.

Gary: I want to go further here in exploring the dynamics of individual, family, and systemic burnout. People in comas are simultaneously individuals and roles in a family and cultural system. Families have a tendency to fix roles even when someone isn't in an extreme space like a coma. There is often the sick one, the caretaker, the good one, and a troublemaker, an alcoholic, or a codependent one. We tend to forget that these are not all of who we are but only a part of ourselves that has been locked into a family system. When someone is in coma, the role of the one who needs care and the caregiver tend to become fixed and rigid. Families I work with will tell me it has been a year or more since they took a break from being at their loved one's bedside. Although being so devoted is highly admirable, the other side of this is that I have worked with so many people in families who have developed physical symptoms since their loved one went into coma. On a causal level, we could say that such high levels of stress cause symptoms. However, I think there is something much more complex and interesting going

Exercise 7.1
Coping with Burnout

1. Make yourself comfortable. Sit back and relax and notice how it feels to be yourself right now.
2. If you are feeling burned out, explore the experience with curiosity. If you don't feel burned out in the moment, remember a time when you had felt overwhelmed, fatigued, distressed, or numbed out.
3. How does that experience feel emotionally, mentally, and in your body? Is it lethargy, "brain freeze," heaviness, emptiness, anxiety, panic, or something else? Uncover that experience with an open mind.
4. Breathe into it and let it engulf you. Give it space and let it move you at its own pace and timing. Become the burnout experience.
5. Explore its way of relating, living, doctoring, helping. Discover its energetic quality. If you want, you can draw a quick energy sketch that captures the essential quality that burnout has for you.
6. Next ask yourself who in you needs this medicine. Who needs burnout? What part of you is the experience of burnout meant for?
7. Let both parts speak and have a dialogue about their values and motivations.

on. The symptoms are reminders that as a family member, you still have a body that has needs and you need to somehow carry on. Frequently the caregivers' symptoms are so severe that I have to work on the family members as well as with the person in coma.

FREEDOM FROM FIXED ROLES

As I mentioned before, one of the exercises I often do with families is I have them imagine they are in a coma. The almost universal response is that people don't want to get up off the floor from this state. It is restful, peaceful, and they love the focus and attention of us helping them unfold this state. This is a first important step toward experiencing what it is like to be out of the caretaker role. Another important step is to then structure in time out of their caretaker role; for example, I have negotiated with many caregivers that they will take one weekend off a month to nurture themselves. Some of this just involves giving information to the family, telling them that burnout is almost universal and preventable, and then helping each individual do what they need to do to take care of themselves. It also helps to name a phenomenon similar to survival guilt, if it is happening. Many people feel that if they identify their loved one as suffering, they then must suffer with them, and they don't allow themselves to enjoy life. Sometimes this is unconsciously translated into a belief that the family members don't have the right to be well if the patient isn't well. Of course with detachment we can see just the opposite. Being a caregiver in a situation like this may go on for months or even years. It is rarely a sprint race, more like a marathon, and people need to know how to take care of themselves and to have permission to do this. In my Coma Work, with families I have helped with back injuries, falls, high blood pressure, flu, heart issues, and lung issues; often the symptoms of the family seem more intense than those of the coma patient.

Until now I have been referring mostly to the outer demands of time, of juggling other parts of one's life with all this caregiving. However, there are also the inner demands of all the emotions we go through when a loved one is in a coma, which also create stress and burnout. I have seen everything from the deepest grief of a parent for a child, to a child glad that his mom was in a coma and dying, and he couldn't wait for her death to come. People need help processing these emotions. They are so often wracked by guilt. Almost everyone thinks they could have done something to prevent the coma, or that they could have been kinder to the person before the coma. People have survivor guilt. They blame themselves for being free to run around in conscious states while their loved ones are in the coma. Many times the love that was never fully expressed comes forward. There is also so much grief for the loss of the person the way they used to be. There is a tremendous range here, from people who feel they can actually relate better to the person in coma, to the wife or husband who feels their partner is suddenly gone and can't relate to them at all in coma. In the background is often anger that this happened, anger at God, at the hospital and doctors, and at the person for being in the coma. That is such an irrational feeling, yet it can very much be present. The job of the coma worker is to help family members process these feelings; we encourage them to feel their feelings without judging them and to express them rather than just being dominated by their feelings. No two relationships are exactly alike. They are mixtures of love, attachment, hate, detachment, fear, jealousy, competition, revenge, attraction, sexuality, spirituality, and every other possible sense of connection and emotion. Coma tends to amplify these feelings. We are suddenly with that person many hours a day. Also being close to death tends to strip away the extra, the superficial, the unsaid and unfelt. For us to be there for the coma person, we need to be able to process our own emotions or they can be so overwhelming we can be swamped and ineffective.

BURNOUT OF THE COMA WORKER

About three years ago, I began to burn out on doing Coma Work. I began to study myself because I thought if I learned why I was burning out, I might be able to help others to prevent and move past burnout. The central factor I found behind my burnout was the belief system that I had to do everything possible to help my clients get better. I had to be in a *work as hard as possible* head and body space. Even though my deepest beliefs are that I trust and follow nature when working with a coma patient, this more ordinary human part of me feels connected to and compassion for the demands and wishes of the family. The burnout started to develop after I had a series of successes with helping people who had been given no chance of returning, to come out of coma. In a way, it is a bit like betting on a horse race and picking a winner the first three times. Suddenly winning becomes something like an addiction that can't be escaped. My success addicted me to this work to some degree. For a while I became attached and one-sided toward the person coming out of coma. I stopped just being a coma worker and became a coma rescuer.

The more I worked on myself, the more this began to change. I learned that burnout is not such a horrible state to be in. Without burning out a bit, how could I find out how I am pushing the river, swimming upstream, overdoing when it isn't helpful or called for, and therefore find that I am out of harmony with my clients and myself? Arnold Mindell has often said that we should be generous and happy with ourselves when we discover we are off the path, as that is such a big step toward following the path. As my real estate agent once told me, "Gary, I am showing you first what you don't want so you will know from this what you do want." Burnout is a teacher and a message carrier. Its message to me was "Gary, you are too attached to making things work." I started to follow my body and let myself sit when I was tired, work when I was energized, and eat when I was hungry. When traveling with a coma patient and his or her family, I would work maybe five hours a day instead of eight. Rather than always working for four days, sometimes just one was enough. I saw myself as a facilitator, rather than a rescue person. I was there to facilitate the next step in the coma person's journey, whether that led to waking up, partial waking up, staying stuck, or death. I began to realize that in following my own body, I was modeling something for both the coma patient and their family. I always start by telling the coma patients to follow themselves and nature, but if I don't practice what I preach, it is a double standard and I give the double message to follow nature even though I don't! So for the coma worker to congruently be in touch with and follow his or her own body process is a crucial step in breaking these addictions to roles. People would often say to me, "Gary, you have so much energy as you work on these people," but I needed to tell them that my energy is dependent on following myself and nature and not just guilt and obligation or even love. Love can be full of freedom or it can bind you to a situation and a role, and I know I have this belief (or prejudice!) that the more freedom there is present, the more love blossoms.

Burnout tells me that the essential Me, the Gary, is being used up; I need to go and connect with nature, with the Earth, and all the energy that is available as I ground myself. Being more conscious is a privilege that I want to use for the benefit of my client. The more I can be my whole self, the more I can help my clients and their families to be their whole selves and step out of the roles that they are stuck playing. As soon as I feel my whole self, I can feel how my process is connected to my clients. We are growing together, sharing issues together, and developing together. It is no longer just me giving, but rather our energies are dancing together. I am growing as my client is growing. I will say more about this in the next chapter, but I mention it here because one of the keys to working with burnout is to realize I am also getting all kinds of personal growth out of this experience, and our growth is somehow connected. Every issue that my clients have had, including bringing forth their introversion, their meditative side, their wild fighter, their love and their sexuality, their rage, their vulnerability, and their determination to live the life they want and not the one others want or expect of them—I am all of these and it is so much more energizing to feel we are growing together than that I am rescuing them from being thrown into the pit of coma.

In Process Work, we talk about the little you and the BIG YOU.[3] The little you is the ordinary person, with all your polarities, conflicts, troubles, and limitations. The BIG YOU is the sum of all of your parts together and the unity and power and mystery this connects you to. One definition of burnout is that when I come from my ordinary personality, I am limited, and will therefore run out of steam, but I have another part of me that is connected to something infinite and can no more burn out than the sun can. Eventually it will of course, but the sun has an almost infinite level of energy. Our work is to help connect the coma person to this infinite level. I am convinced that part of what is behind coma is an attempt to get past the limited self and move toward some experience of this BIG YOU. Person after person who comes back from near-death experiences talks about an encounter with something bigger and more universal than themselves. By connecting with this BIG YOU part of myself, I model and join the client at this universal spot. One of my goals of being a coma worker is to make the journey less lonely, and the more people I feel can join me in this state, the less I am burned out, and the less the client and their family will be, too.

BURNOUT AND THE MEDICAL SYSTEM

Pierre has already covered this topic, but it is important to mention that all of the principles I have mentioned in relation to family members also apply within the medical system. So many medical practitioners are burning out. I have heard so many express their sense of failure in dealing with coma patients whom they could not save or bring back. Doctors are often pushed far beyond their body limits. One of the central positions of most healing professions is to separate ourselves from the clients emotionally and to recognize the differences between us and them, and to keep this barrier, this boundary of difference very clear. This is one way to protect ourselves from being overwhelmed and over-attached. Unfortunately it also cuts medical people off from this sense of entanglement, of oneness, of how their personal development and the client's are related. A medical system that views change as "when Sadie can sit up and play cards again" as one doctor told me, sets people up for hopelessness and despair. If the only criterion for success is to return to a prior state of consciousness, we risk skipping over so many little moments of transformation in any direction, toward consciousness, or toward death.

PICKING UP NEGATIVE FEELINGS FROM YOUR CLIENT

One of the big concerns many practitioners have is that they might actually pick up something like a negative emotion from their client. Many therapists describe this as part of burnout. Working with too many depressed clients can lead to something like a depression. If you are a neurologist, it may be that working with too many clients who seem hopeless may lead to your being hopeless. In traditional cultures, shamans have always feared picking up some kind of negative energy, or having negative energy thrown at them. Much illness is seen as this invasion of negative energy. This fear can be of enemies, especially people who are jealous of you, but also some shamans become sick working on someone else. From a Process Work standpoint, we can only pick up what we need for our own process.

If I am working with a coma patient and I develop a headache in the same spot where the person was injured when they went into coma, then I probably have some common dreamlike process going on with that person. When I am working I constantly scan my body, and if a new or more intense pain or symptom pops up, I explore it. There are many Process Work inner work methods for working with the energy of anything we may have "picked up." If I only have a short time to do this while working with a client, I use one of two main methods. First I go inside, feel the symptom more, and intuitively guess at what meaning or direction this symptom has for me. Sometimes that is enough for the symptom to clear. This is like waking up after a dream and then simply sitting and meditating on the dream until the meaning pops in. If this clears the symptom from that part of my body, my work is at least momentarily done. If not, I might go back into the symptom and try to amplify it even more, to feel or experience it more. I would then track what happens next and try to take this symptom into different channels of experience, such as vision, sound, movement, relationship, feeling, and relationship to the world and to the spiritual realms. I would then go back and see if this changed the symptom.

The more we practice, the quicker these symptoms move. For example, let's say I start to get a headache when working on a client. I know she has a lot of head issues from her head injury. I go inside and feel my headache. I make an intuitive guess that I have sadness around this whole thing. I go inside and feel my sadness for a moment, and the headache mostly disappears. Then I try expressing the headache in movement. I clench my fists to represent the tension in my head. I take a minute to let my fists express the frustration I am carrying. I check in with my headache, and the pain is gone. My work is temporarily over for me, but I then think of my client and how my headache and her process might be connected. Maybe then I go over and help her to make fists and see what kind of action and response I receive doing this. Processing what comes up prevents burnout. There is also a moment in a process to not process, but to put one's feet up and just breathe. The more we work with ourselves and know ourselves, the more we know how to recognize the internal and relationship signals that tell us when it is time to process, and when it is time to relax.

Chapter 8

Coma as Our Teacher

Working with coma patients teaches us so much about living and dying. This chapter focuses on the coma patient as a teacher of the value of life and about the diversity of all states of consciousness. Coma patients teach all of us about being in internal states. Coma Work also makes us much more aware in the realm of touch, and this can be applied to our work with patients and to how we touch our friends and loved ones. The chapter ends by discussing how Coma Work wakes us up to a whole world of nonverbal signals in our communication, self-expression, and relationships.

Coma Work skills allow us to validate our own subtle altered states and times of reduced cognitive functioning. Getting acquainted with these different states of consciousness on a daily basis is powerful preventive medicine. Following our flow of consciousness as it moves from alertness to dreaming and empty mind is a powerful tool that helps us cope with everyday reality and makes our lives more meaningful. Familiarity with these states allows us to relate to our patients, clients, and loved ones as they experience the changes that come with coma, illness, and aging.

Gary: During a conversation with our publisher about this book, she suggested we write about how working with coma patients had changed us as people. At first I was perplexed, and then I was fascinated by this perspective on the field of Coma Work, as previously I have always focused on what I am doing for and with the coma patient. In this chapter, I share some of my thinking about how Coma Work is transforming and awakening me.

THE LITTLE ENGINE THAT COULD

When I work with coma patients, my overriding experience is that of thankfulness for the body that I have. At 54, everything works pretty well. I am also constantly in awe of two basic principles of the brain. The first is how complex the brain is and how much I take it for granted that; for example, when I want to change shirts, my brain tells my hands exactly what to do and it happens. Working with people with brain injuries makes me realize how often I ignore the miracle of the working brain. I am now more careful with bike helmets, ski helmets, and other preventive measures, knowing that, with the brain, it is much easier to prevent than to heal, and I am just loving and appreciating my brain as it functions so well. The second basic principle that I have learned is that this amazing center of intelligence that we have is also incredibly intuitively wise about how to repair itself, if we can only support this happening. So my Coma Work makes me bow in awe to the power of the brain to heal itself.

I have learned from this ability of the brain to heal itself, to stop accepting what consensus reality says is possible and what isn't. About a third of the people I have worked with, of whom are given less than 5 percent chance of recovery, have recovered to the point of being able to communicate verbally. Before Coma Work, I would often get to challenging places in my life where someone would say that something was impossible, and I would believe them. When I was a child, my parents, who were generally wonderful people, sometimes would, out of their more conservative natures, tell me I couldn't do something; it was too big a dream and I was too little. Yet some part of me believed and knew that there was another realm of possibility, of dreams and dream-like experiences. My favorite childhood book was *The Little Engine that Could*, which is about a big train and a little train. The fancy, shiny, big train took toys over the mountains to the children, but the little train was only used around the train yard. One day the big train broke down, and there was no way to get the toys to the children. The little train said that it could do it, but everyone laughed and said, "Impossible!" But the little train huffed and puffed and kept saying, "I think I can, I think I can," and it made it over the mountain. For me, the big train has often been consensus reality, but the little train was a dream train, and it had powers that were often unseen and yet ready to be brought forward at the right moment.

None of my coma patients who have come out of coma and made significant recoveries were given any chance of recovery, according to mainstream medical standards. Yet I often saw that little engine puffing and huffing, and I would puff and huff with it until the person came back. I have learned to face other challenges in the same way. Sometimes when I get injured physically, particularly in Aikido, I think I am going to be out for weeks, but then that little train in me goes to work on the symptom and I am most often better in a few days or less. Even though the legal system often tells me our fight is hopeless, I am currently facing a legal challenge around a foster daughter I have taken on with my partner, Sharon, to prevent her being sent back to her family, to whom she doesn't want to return. Coma patients have taught me that nothing is impossible when we bring in the powers of our whole selves. Coma patients inoculate us against being hypnotized into believing that we are only limited, small beings. The little engine is connected to the whole universe. We are enormous, powerful people with unbelievable potential energy for all kinds of uses. If my coma patient, who was hit by a car, then attacked with a knife, left for dead on the streets, and written off as dead by the hospital, can come back and go to college, then I can see something heroic in front of me that models for all of us our ability to reach deep inside ourselves and to go beyond our perceived limits.

These experiences also change my view of the medical model. If the brain injured people I work with so often defy conventional views about illness and injury, this must also be true about other aspects of our bodies and their symptoms, and this certainly goes along with my experiences working with clients with all kinds of body symptoms. With Process Work interactions supporting medical interventions, it is rare that my clients ever have the exact outcomes that their doctors predict for them. For example, if I look at my clients over the years who had terminal cancer, most of those I worked with lived on average at least twice as long as they were told they would. All of this needs further research, but the main principle here is the one I learned from my coma patients more than any other clients, which is that the body is a dreaming, mysterious temple that doesn't just follow principles of mechanics and matter, and that as we learn to open up to what is "wrong" with our bodies as a process, rather than just a fixed condition, then there are many possible outcomes, not just the medically defined ones.

COMA PATIENTS AS MEDITATION MASTERS

There are so many different kinds of coma patients, distinguished not only by the kind of coma and the circumstances of the coma, but also by who that person is now and who they were before the coma. One major experience in comas is that some people seem to be in deep meditation. In such a busy, extroverted world, they are the "City Shadows," carrying the most marginalized, cast-off parts of society, which is why when I sometimes have family members of coma patients go inside themselves and imagine that they are in a coma, they are shocked at the relief they experience. They are also relieved to be able to eventually come out of their imagined comas, but still the momentary state is often blissful.

I was in Switzerland once and was asked to work with John who was in a coma. I walked in and saw a relatively young man who had had a stroke. Without knowing anything about him, I mentioned how relaxed his body was, that he looked like he was on a vacation. I began to ask about his life. John was a restaurant owner. He worked 14 hour days, seven days a week, and hadn't taken a holiday in years. Now John looked like he was having a long overdue rest and was just being—not doing. I asked several people who came in for their impressions of him during this coma, including medical staff, and nuns who came in, as it was a religious-based hospital. They all said how peaceful John looked now and had for much of the time in his coma. I talked to John about taking a break, going inside, getting to slow down and feel and be vegetative and meditative. He gave me great feedback, took a big breath, and relaxed even more.

Linette was an elderly woman who had had a stroke. When I first walked into the room to meet her, I was struck by how she held herself; I said, "It was like sitting with Buddha." I tried a lot of more related interventions, moving her body, touching her, talking with her, trying different relationship interventions with her huge family. But there was no feedback to anything. Suddenly I realized that I am so extroverted at times that I was expecting her to meet me in my world. I started to meditate and kept meditating with her for a long time. Then I suddenly got this idea to count and see if I could get her to open her eyes on a certain count, "One, two, three, four, five, six, seven, eight." On eight, her eyes popped open, then closed. "One, two, three, four, five, six, seven, eight," her eyes opened again. I tried to match the counting to her breath. She was meditating, and she was teaching me to be more meditative. We went on like this for hours. At one point she had about 15 family members packed into her room trying to relate to her, but Linette just meditated. If anyone wanted to be with her, it was through meditation that they could enter her space. This was in contrast to others; for example, Steve, who wrestled with me, grunted, and threw fits while in a coma, or Lisa who curled up into my arms when I first touched her. They were great teachers of rough and gentle contact. Some people in comatose states are very related, but many are there to do their inner work and are teachers of the importance of this. I have to remember this as a coma worker, that I am there to facilitate their internal process, and in doing this I have to relate to my own internal process. I don't want to polarize more and more and be the external voice pushing people deeper into their internal space, but I must instead find my own internal space, and meet them from there.

When I walk into the room, the family is often full of expectations, no matter what I do to try and reduce expectations. Often they may have paid out lots of money to bring me to their country, or to wherever they are in the United States, to their loved one. I can be totally caught up in all of this pressure. In many cases, we are seen as the last hope. How do I keep my center and meditate under all this pressure? How do I avoid just becoming the force trying to pull the person out of coma and provoking resistance in doing this? First, I rely on my training; second, I let the coma person remind me what it is like to be inside, and I follow what is inside and for a few moments I am able to ignore the pressures by being unrelated to the outside. I am so naturally in relationship that the coma person's freedom not to follow what is asked on the outside is a great reminder for me. This freedom to be inner-directed and at times to ignore outside pressures has been taught to me over and over again by the coma patient meditation masters.

Process-oriented Psychology has a unique style of meditation. In most other meditative approaches, we focus only on whatever we are using to take us out of our ordinary awareness, for example, the breath. We develop the watcher, the witness. In Process Work we also do this, but we then apply this awareness, which we call Process Mind, to what is coming up. A traditional meditator would notice a thought or feeling or image or whatever came up, and then let it pass. In Process Work, we might do this, but we might also use this centered place to enter into whatever came up, and work with it. So if I am meditating and I suddenly have an image of a fire, I might step in and become that fire, and then step out and see how that fire and the ordinary Gary—the one I think of as Gary—are one, and make up my BIG YOU that is bigger than the sum of all of my parts. I might move and breathe like that fire, and then I ask myself where I need more of that in my life. This is what I see we have to teach the coma meditation masters. Many of them seem to really have mastered how to stay inside and very close to themselves. However, they seem not to know what to do with the kinds of experiences they are having. My job is to help them learn how to climb into these experiences, how to surf them, swim them, ride them like a horse, and fly with them as if on the wings of a giant bird. This seems to be very helpful to these states. The best learning situations are where teacher and student are fluid roles that we can all occupy. In working with coma patients, I am both: I am a student at one moment and a teacher at another.

In Process Work, we help people go deeper beyond the places where they are stuck. We go into deeper and deeper states of awareness to a place where, for example, I am not only my limited consciousness of Gary or even the bigger consciousness of Gary I might have if I have worked on my dreams and dreamlike experience, but rather I am part of a greater consciousness that goes beyond just me. This consciousness is non-local, and connects me directly with the Earth and with the cosmos. If I am aware that I am not just Gary but also the ocean, or the stars, I have a different kind of awareness process that helps me to perceive who I am and what life is from a very different perspective than my ordinary consciousness. In Process Work we call this deeper, sentient-based awareness *Process Mind*.

When I work with coma patients, they teach me about this non-locality principle. I often ask them if they are in the sky or whether they are in the ocean now, or if they are a whale. I have had amazing feedback to these kinds of inquiries. In this way, they are enlightenment teachers, teaching me that my consciousness tends to get very attached to my limited identity of Gary. Going into a coma may be an attempt to connect to this Process Mind. However, when I am working with a coma patient, they are teaching me how to get into these states without my needing to be in a coma or on drugs. As I learn to explore these states, I am discovering how healing they can be for mind, body, and spirit. When I connect with my coma patients at this level of Process Mind, miraculous changes may occur (see Chapter 6 for more on this level of the work).

COMA WORK AS TOUCH AND TANTRIC TEACHER

I have always liked touching people. I trained for awhile in various bodywork techniques including acupressure, Traeger, and Swedish massage, and with other Process Workers I have helped to develop various approaches to a more Process-oriented body work. I also studied massage partially to be a better lover with my sexual partners. However, Coma Work, more than any other experience, trained me in how to touch someone. Why? Because there is no verbal feedback, so you have to go with nonverbal feedback and your own intuition. We must develop sensitivity to the slightest reactions. How many of us when we are giv-ing a massage notice how the person's breath, skin color, or muscle tone indicates to us exactly how he or she wants to be touched? I grew up in a very verbal culture, so to develop this sensitivity, this inner quietness and communication that comes through my hands, was an incredible learning for me. In my work as a sex therapist, many couples com-plained that they have no communication, verbal or nonverbal, around their sex life. I have worked with so many people who have told me sto-ries about how they felt their partner never touched them in the way they wanted to be touched or even approached this realm of touch. Now I can teach people how to pick up on the most minimal cues and become much more sensitive lovers.

Learning how to be sensitive to nonverbal feedback is applicable far beyond touch and sexuality. All of our communication would improve if we paid attention to the feedback that is coming to us. Also, the more we can notice feedback from other people, the more we begin to notice our own internal signals. For example, I work with many athletes whose injuries come from their refusal to listen to their own bodies. We are trained to make the doctors the experts about our bodies, rather than to use them as consultants and developing our own expertise about our bodies by noticing and following our own feedback.

Coma Work wakes me up to all of this. It is paradoxical that people in the most far away, most deeply withdrawn states are such effective awakeners of sensitivity in others. Maybe part of the meaning of so many people going into these states is that they are there partially to wake themselves up, but also to wake us all up. In an extroverted, verbal, constantly in-touch society, those in coma reflect a parallel world that we can all learn from and integrate into our daily lives. We can learn to move fluidly between inner and outer, extroverted and quiet, related and nonrelated states. Working with coma patients is much more fun, successful, and sustainable for Coma Workers if we realize that we are growing together, client and patient, awakening to the world of living and integrating our altered and extreme states of conscious-ness. It isn't just the coma person who has trouble moving fluidly in and out of these states; it is all of us. We are all learning together.

Pierre: When we experience coma and altered states, and in general, when our brains are not working as we would like them to, we are con-fronted with a process that challenges our identity and sense of self. Coma itself is still relatively rare but we all go through various stages of changed consciousness all the time. When we wake up in the morning we go through a radical process of transitioning from unconsciousness or a dream state to our usual functioning state of mind. Most of the time we pay little attention to that shift in awareness and immediately forget the sleep state. We ready ourselves to face the challenges of daily wakeful living. Later in the evening we might drink some alcohol or unwind in front of the TV set and enjoy a more relaxed and dreamy state.

When we get burned out from our work load or get a flu we are forced to rejoin alternate states of consciousness. But rarely do we explore these states. On the contrary, we usually marginalize them in favor of our consensual wakeful states. Most of us define reality from the experience we have while being awake and alert and we disavow altered states of consciousness from contributing to what we call "real" experiences.

By putting so much emphasis on consensual wakeful states, we reject a big part of who we are. That is also a reason why addictions are so popular—because, through them, we are attempting to re-connect with an alternate dreaming reality. Connecting to processes that expand our awareness of reality keeps us in touch with our dreaming bodies. If you are tired and force yourself to keep going, or if you drink coffee, repress the tiredness, and pursue your activities as if nothing had happened, then later the tiredness will work on you and have its long-term effects. If instead you try to move with the flow of your process and step into the experience of tiredness you might experience yourself going inside into a peaceful state. Instead of feeling tired, you might feel as if time had slowed down and you might find yourself going at a slower pace. Resisting nature and the natural changes in consciousness is something that we all have learned to do to function in life. Nevertheless, this marginalization process might also be a cause of illness and disease. Staying in touch with our bodies and their subtle changes in energy might be good preventative medicine.

In addition, if you learn to follow your body's process and allow yourself to experience your various natural altered states of consciousness you might be able to tune yourself into subtle sentient experiences that can be very creative and meaningful from a spiritual viewpoint. The changes that come with aging, for example, low energy and memory loss, are problems only when seen from a viewpoint that emphasizes alertness and wakefulness. From a viewpoint of allowing the dreaming process of your bodies to unfold, the symptoms of aging become a path toward wholeness. Individual memories and identities fade to make space for dreamlike experiences that unite us with alternate dreaming realities.

Before my mother died after a long illness with cancer, she entered a world of silence and reduced communication. She stopped relating to us, her children, though she continued to answer the nurses' questions about her pain or comfort levels. I felt she had left her role as a parent and gone into a dreaming state. At that time I wasn't very aware of my own dreaming and kept feeling hurt for the interrupted communication and relationship. I wish I had been more aware of my own fixation about relating to her in consensual-reality terms. Using our own dreaming processes allows us to stay more related to our loved ones when they go through transitional processes in death and dying. Also if as health professionals we were more aware of our own altered states we might gain a different understanding of delusional and demented processes. Learning to experience our clients and patients in these states as powerful dreamers will change our ability to relate to them and help family members to understand their loved ones.

In general, our current medical ethics and best practices originate from consensus reality frameworks. From this vantage point we and our patients have symptoms that need cure and palliation. Medication will calm our clients' agitation and our own discomfort with the unknown of our unconscious and its dreamlike powers. However, in my personal experience agitation often develops because of a communication breakdown between us and our dreaming patients. Many of my patients have calmed down once I joined them in their dreaming experience. The disturbing sounds and body movements they were making were connected with inner visual experiences and once I supported them using Coma Work skills the disturbing "symptoms" became powerful processes that relieved the patient.

Elderly people often develop a sense of suspicion and anxiety which can progress to full paranoia. As health care professionals we are trained to address these issues with behavioral plans that aim to reduce and control these pathological behaviors. We are taught to confront our patients' disturbing behaviors and help them reclaim their previous and more "normal" perspective on reality. We often deny their experiences in the hope of giving them a renewed sense of reality and "normality" and improve their ability to cope with and adjust to their declining health and the aging process. In the elderly memory loss, cognitive impairments, anxiety, and suspicion are clearly interrelated and need coordinated treatment. From a mainstream view our clients' suspicion and paranoia might appear unfounded and difficult to understand. On the other hand, if we validate their experiences and allow ourselves to join their dreaming reality, we might discover that our clients' suspicion is not only based on cognitive changes but may also reflect unresolved relationship issues or other meaningful processes.

Chapter 9

Relating to the Hospital, Health Care Team, and Family

Cultural and philosophical clashes are an intrinsic part of treating individuals in coma. Here we describe and explain how to facilitate conflicts generated by these life and death issues, between families and health care teams, between individual members of the care teams, and within families themselves, and offer guidance on working with your own and others' skepticism and hopelessness.

UNCERTAINTY AND EXPERTISE

Pierre: In previous chapters we have explored coma and altered states from an individual and relationship angle. We have looked at health and healing and at ways to process burnout. In this chapter we discuss systemic aspects of Coma Work and how cultural views affect relationships in care teams and between care teams, patients, and family members. One factor that strongly influences the relationships between health professionals and "lay" sick people and their families is the predominating focus of the doctors and medical care teams on self-confidence and expertise. While knowledge and expertise are unquestionably essential for good medical practice, the myth of the infallible and invulnerable doctor helps create an unrealistic expectation and widens the gap between doctors and patients. Our fallibility and its consequences are well documented—medical errors and iatrogenic complications are a significant source of morbidity, mortality, and medical costs. In 2000, members of a presidential task force estimated that the cost (lost income, disability, and health care costs) associated with these errors could be as much as $29 billion annually. That same year the Institute of Medicine released a historic report, "To Err Is Human: Building a Safer Health System."[1] The authors concluded that 44,000 to 98,000 people die each year as a result of errors during hospitalization. The Hippocratic Oath that all doctors take to practice medicine ethically and "first, do no harm" received a new systemic dimension. The report begins with an acknowledgment of the inherent dangers in medicine and of the fallibility of every health professional. It continues with the need to ensure a humane environment for medical practice that allows clinicians to be vulnerable. Professionalism and expertise are extremely relevant for an effective medicine. We want better and more proficient doctors. In addition to mastering the hard technical skills, doctors and all health professionals also need to become relationship experts. This includes diversity awareness, cultural competence, and knowledge of rank and power dynamics, as well as an understanding of the softer emotional skills. In chronic care management, as a helper you are a companion to the diseased and their families, you accompany them on their journey to live meaningful lives with their illnesses.

The strong orientation of today's medical practice toward excellence, reducing errors, and cost effectiveness is pertinent to advancing medicine. Evidence-based medicine and best practice treatment schemes are important attempts at improving health care and lowering costs. In medicine the prevailing relational model is based on informed consent and strives for the ideal of two people capable of mature, responsible judgment. The foundation of this therapeutic alliance lies in a rational contract between the doctor and patient. This model encourages patient emancipation and autonomy and counterbalances the previously paternalistic attitude of many doctors and health professionals. Unfortunately it also marginalizes the understanding that all of us, patients and professionals, are also psychological beings with unconscious and irrational value judgments and feelings. The therapeutic alliance may be distorted by the sometimes unconscious wishes and expectations of the patient and the doctor. Communication between doctors and patients occurs in social, psychological, and emotional contexts that reflect the personalities of those involved. The complex and dynamic interactions between doctors and patients take place in a social, cultural, and ethical field in which uncertainty and subjectivity reign.

All of us sense ourselves both as an object, as a person with a "mechanical" body we can use, and as an experiencing subject, a person who sets a goal and tries to achieve it. Today's mainstream medicine sees the body mainly as an object—an instrument that breaks down and needs to be fixed. Biomedicine inherited this fundamentally diminishing model of the body from the scientific view that matter, including the human body, is of its nature spiritless—an insentient thing. As patients we all feel the bias of this thinking; not only does our subjective testimony become alienated, but our bodily knowledge as a whole is also marginalized.

The classic scientific formulation that only reason and objectivism are valid concepts needs to be extended to include an understanding that the human psyche is part of the living system and that the objective cannot function without the subjective. Our communication must address the subjective as well as the objective aspects of the relationship between clinician and patient. In objective medicine things operate by cause and effect, but not so in the world of relationship. Relationship interactions take place in a complex field of forces (contextual, psychological, social, and cultural) and are thus governed by an uncertainty principle. Social and cultural beliefs and values, and individual feelings and goals, create an atmospheric field in which there is a prospective uncertainty as to the outcome of any given relationship interaction. The dynamic interactions among these biological, physical, social, cultural, ethical, and emotional elements are unpredictable, as are the outcomes. In communication the result of our individual observations will not be completely objective but will reflect the facets of the many processes involved. Knowledge and understanding of communication and relationship signals (for example, rank signals) and the conceptual and cultural metaphors people live by facilitate a process awareness and interpersonal understanding. It helps us to tolerate the uncertainty and negotiate meaning.

Arnold Mindell[2] describes various ways in which power may be experienced. He differentiates between six distinct dimensions of personal power and rank: social, educational, psychological, relational, transpersonal or spiritual, and contextual. His definition of rank includes social dynamics such as marginalization and oppression based on class, gender, race, and sexual orientation, and internalized processes of handling inner diversity, self-love, and self-esteem. As individuals our perception of our rank and our marginalization history can contribute to feelings of powerlessness and can influence our sense of a coherent and meaningful life. Social rank issues also affect our health-related behaviors and lead to worse health outcomes.[3] In the clinician/caregiver-patient relationship, rank plays an important role. The helper has more rank than the one receiving help. Being healthy and not being injured or disabled comes with rank, too. If you recall Chris's story, he was dealing with several rank issues that contributed to his relationship problems. His healthy wife had

difficulties tolerating his hopelessness and depression. He was also struggling with an internalized sense of oppression between his old healthy self
and the new self that was facing significant physical and cognitive impair-
ment. In Cenan's case, the whole care team had difficulties opening up to
culturally diverse communication styles.

One-sided expertise and objectivity alienate health professionals from
their patients and their families. They widen the rank and power differential and contribute to communication blocks. Patients have power,
too. As health care professionals we instinctively know that, were we to
make a mistake, the patient would have many advocates and the media
on his or her side all seeking retribution. The patients and their families
rely on us and we need to use our rank with awareness. Good use of
our rank includes opening ourselves up to our uncertainty and vulnerability. When I helped Chris's wife to do that, it changed their relationship dynamic and resolved some of their conflicts.

As health care professionals much of our training is premised on the
erroneous idea that we can treat our patients from an uninvolved neutral and objective position. Subjective experiences on both sides get disenfranchised in this process, both those doing the caring and those
being cared for. As Susan Griffin says, "Any illness can be read as a
metaphor of the soul. But it is not just one soul that lies in the balance.
Illness of every kind holds up a mirror to society."[4] Scientist, healer,
patient, family member, and society are not only separate independent
systems. We are also all inseparably linked with one another. The entire
knowledge of human experience and emotions is in everyone. As wit-
nesses of, and listeners to, illness narratives, we are drawing on our ability to share and partake in the experience. They are stories we will all
hear and experience and, as they move through our bodies, they have
the power to change us all.

PROPOSAL FOR A RELATIONSHIP MEDICINE

In my opinion, what is missing in the medical world is a relationship-
and community-based medicine and way of thinking, which include
the systemic dimensions of health and illness. We all make huge efforts to
become competent and qualified in our professional fields. To do justice
to our dual role as experts and human companions, we also need to
become relationship experts, too. Most health care professionals believe
that the ability to feel for their patients is an important dimension
of treatment, but the relationship training lags behind the training in
the hard technical skills. Sometimes we will be asked to step into the role

of a detached scientist or technician, but at other times we will have to take on the role of an empathic healer or an empowering adult educator, who can be a resource for the patient's own healing efforts. Our lack of knowledge about the relevance of cultural metaphors in relationship such as rank can sometimes cause symptoms to worsen and become chronic. I am convinced that it is time to liberate disease from its individual context and incorporate the social dimension into our treatment practices. Alongside technical development, new relationship awareness must also be integrated into the therapeutic alliance.

Relationship medicine stresses the importance and primacy of the clinician-patient *relationship*. Satisfaction for both and the degree of patient compliance with treatment plans are directly related to the quality of their relationship. Kaplan[5] showed that patients tended to leave doctors who failed to involve them in decisions. Furthermore, I believe that adequate participation in decision making and adherence to treatment plans requires that as clinicians we develop an awareness of the experiential diversity that our patients bring into the relationship.

Cultural and social issues can no longer be left out of the discussion about good doctor-patient relationships. Therapists and physicians are responsible for more democratic relationships. The integration of an adult education paradigm will lead to an attitude of seeing the relationship as a form of learning community, where people are interested in each person's individual cultural and experiential background. This new relational model will help overcome power differentials between clinician and patient.

One possible way to understand the dynamics of clinician and client's social background is to discuss our various levels of rank and privilege. Every intervention could then follow the flow of the patient's inner and worldly stories. I imagine a new relationship awareness where the health care provider tries to form an alliance with the client's inner and outer processes. We can then begin to interpret so-called side effects, such as adverse reactions to a drug therapy and lack of compliance from the patient, as a result of our failure to connect with the patient's inner process or as a lack of understanding of their societal circumstances.

Here are some anecdotal examples of the way social processes may influence health. A friend of mine told me how her father, a physician and a highly recognized specialist in his field, used to gossip about rural people who wouldn't go and see a doctor in spite of serious health conditions. We both wondered if people might have absented themselves out of resentment toward the cultural gap between a highly technologized medical system and their simpler lifestyle. Another friend told me how his experienced doctor had been very timid about examining his prostate.

Their shared discomfort about this particular examination was relieving and healing for my friend. We all know how much we appreciate it when we feel met by our peers in our inner experience and inner diversity.[6] In more hierarchical relationships, we all tend to forget that people come with very different life experiences and need to be valued for that.

Another systemic question we need to ask is how we as a society deal with the limitations of financial resources for health care and who provides for what sort of care. Does the medical system have to care for social inequities, the consequences of which might be expressed through symptoms? Social, cultural, and economic factors have just as much, if not more, impact on health than do the quantity and quality of resources being invested in the detection and treatment of illness. It is time we reallocate our scarce resources in a way that recognizes that the health of the population is also affected by the ways in which individuals perceive and structure their collective lives.

Relationship medicine methodology includes societal issues such as rank and privilege and the uncertainty of the many forces influencing the clinician-patient relationship. A relational model based on an uncertainty principle reminds doctors that they operate with incomplete and unknowable data and in the context of many simultaneous subjective states of being. In this context, knowledge is merely a role that can be shared and that coexists with uncertainty, vulnerability, and openness to the unknown. This new model relies more on awareness than on expertise and includes the health care professionals' uncertainty and vulnerability as an important key to an improved relationship.

The internalized medical values of excellence and effectiveness also contribute to a sense of inner oppression for health care professionals. The constant pressure of having to live up to these values and the fact that none of us can ever fully achieve these elitist standards contributes to the high stress levels among medical professionals and may actually create unnecessary errors. Bringing in our uncertainty and vulnerability counteracts these oppressive values and helps establish a healthier environment for both clinicians and patients.

Including cultural and social metaphors in the realm of body symptoms helps to relieve the individual patient's burden—without denying that we all carry some responsibility for our symptoms—and puts the issue in a broader context. We all share the guilt and the beauty of our collective world. Symptoms may have meaning for the individual, but they are also an expression of the entanglement of our world. The widely publicized stories of Terri Schiavo and Rom Houben illustrate this cultural entanglement. These stories engage all of us on an existential level and bring up important ethical issues that affect us all.

Relationship medicine addresses internalized issues of self-acceptance and self-esteem and outer interpersonal and social issues such as positive relations with others, perceived rank, and social status. By including subjective and experiential aspects of our lives, it aims to nurture our sense of a coherent and meaningful world. Maybe in the future health care professionals will be relationship experts, too. Whether they are internists, general practitioners, nurse or nurse practitioners, physical therapists, social workers, or psychologists, they will have a sophisticated view of the relationship between emotions, social environment, and health. Their relationship medicine approach will focus on awareness of these many influences and support the flux of the developing process.

SYSTEMIC ASPECTS OF COMA WORK

When we are caring for individuals in comatose states, we enter into a wide and controversial field that elicits great public debate. Our modern lifestyle and medical advances mean it is likely that increasing numbers of individuals will go through these altered states of consciousness. However, our understanding of altered cognitive and mental processes in remote states of consciousness is still very much in the early stages of development. From a materialistic stance, the question is: How much integrative brain function does it take to create the experience we associate with mind or consciousness? This view conflicts with spiritual beliefs that assign humans an independent soul or mind. The process-oriented paradigm, on the other hand, sees body and mind as two manifestations of the underlying creative force or Process Mind for which people have used various names such as God, spirit, Brahman, pilot wave, etc.

Individual caregivers have diverse beliefs, philosophical ideas, and spiritual views upon which they rely for guidance, decision making, and treatment interventions. Contradicting materialistic and dualistic philosophies hover in the background and influence relationships between policy makers, caregivers, and affected families. As we stated in the introduction to this chapter, cultural and philosophical clashes are an intrinsic part of treating individuals in coma and remote states of consciousness. These conflicts happen between families and health care teams, between individual team members of the care teams, and within families themselves. They are rarely overt but linger in moods and attitudes that may have an impact on the patients' chances of recovery.[7] The prevailing materialistic assumptions within medical teams often create a strong sense of hopelessness. The scenario tends to go like this: based on data from outcome studies, which until now have shown little success in any type of rehabilitative procedures, medical professionals often make poor prognostic statements and transfer patients into nursing homes, where they receive minimal sustenance care. Health insurances base their coverage of rehabilitative interventions on the same prognostic criteria and therefore tend to determine that, if there are no obvious signs of progress toward recovery, further medical interventions are unnecessary. Families are then left hanging without medical or financial support, and they will try to fight for their loved ones who have no voice at all. They will challenge the medical decision making process and demand more interventions. Doctors and other caregivers are then often stuck between wanting to attend to the families' needs and the cost limitations imposed by the health care system. Within families, individual members will hang onto the smallest thread of hope and, for example, search the Internet for support and alternative treatment approaches. Other family members will stand for the more "realistic" views and oppose any complementary interventions. Being hopeless or hopeful, realistic or optimistic, are roles determined by the cultural and contextual field. Some of these roles, depending on the context and who embodies them, have more power and rank and therefore have more impact on the course of the disease process.

Process Work recognizes the validity of the many views and roles and attempts to facilitate the debates or conflicts. It understands the group process as part of the patient's process and uses conflict facilitation methods to move the debate forward. We work with family and care team members and facilitate discussions about what everybody is thinking and feeling. If the atmosphere and the attitudes are supportive, we take it inside the patient's room and look for his or her reactions to the various voices and views. This at times allows us to infer possible directions for further treatment interventions. Working with people in comas, their families, and care teams is complex and occurs within a specific socio-cultural context that has its advantages and limitations. It requires cultural competency in the sense of knowledge of the various social and relationship factors. It also requires awareness of the roots of one's own values, beliefs, biases, and privileges. They are the cornerstone of culturally competent encounters and interpersonal relatedness.

WORKING WITH STAFF

Gary: Pierre has done a wonderful job of describing the possibilities of relationship-based medicine approaches. The relationship that I am now going to focus on is the one between the coma worker and the hospital staff. I have had two very different kinds of experiences relating to staff and relating to administration. In terms of most of the staff, I have found a keen sense of interest and mutual respect for each other's work. It is obvious that I need them and all the life-sustaining functions they provide. Many of the staff workers have expressed interest in my methods, and I have started to train some of the staff at hospitals where I work. Physical therapists, speech therapists, and nurses have shown the most interest. Some neurologists have also been very curious about what I do. In general, I have noticed a kind of mutual respect that happens. They try to stay out of my way and be supportive, and I try to stay out of their way, too. We both know we have important work to do. Often staff have been incredibly supportive and encouraging, because they know that many of the patients we work with have made little progress previously and, out of their dedication to their patients, they want to see all possible help given to them.

I have also been to hospitals where the administration is overtly challenging and suspicious. In some countries, every type of healer comes in and often there are charlatans ready to capitalize on the family's desperation for some kind of magical healing. In situations like this, I know that if I can just be allowed to do my work, staff will almost certainly see changes that make them realize that I am doing work that can be of genuine benefit to their patients. Some will embrace these changes; for others, there could be real hostility to the changes this work brings and the fear that we may not be genuine healers, but only there for the money.

Working with Administrators

With hospital administrators and chief physicians, I have had a different experience. Once I was joking with a colleague about different hospitals I had worked at in Israel. They would name one and I would respond with whether or not I had been thrown out of that hospital. Despite my best efforts to relate to the administration and get permission to work in the hospital, something would always come up. In one hospital, I was allowed to work a few times until the head of the whole unit found out about my work. I had been invited to speak to the entire staff about this work. Afterward, the head of speech therapy who had invited me told me that the chief of all chiefs had heard about my talk and had even attended it. However, since I hadn't asked for his permission, and when I met him, not knowing who he was, I hadn't spent time with him or recognized the importance of relating to him, he was now saying I must leave the hospital immediately without even saying good-bye to my client, as if saying good-bye to someone in coma could hurt them. You can sense my frustration here. However, later on in this section I will describe the meeting I had with him a year later, when I learned and understood what was behind his closed attitude. It wasn't personal to me, but about where he was at in his life and career. Another time I was given permission to work by the head doctor of the hospital, but the next day, when a different doctor was acting as head, I was told to leave.

I learned a great deal about how to work on relationships with administration from these experiences. The main quality to bring forward is compassion and understanding for the difficult circumstances the systems are operating in and all the competing pressures they are under from family, physicians, insurance companies, and others. A new paradigm challenges the ways these systems have functioned for a long period of time. It has taken me years to develop more compassion for that voice that says, "Whatever you offer, we don't need it and don't want it!" Now I would say, "My goodness, I know where you are coming from. I have increasingly explored where my own belief systems are fixed and habitual, and where I have benefited so much from those belief systems in the past it is hard to open to changing to something, even if it may work better and serve me and my clients' needs more than my present system. Sometimes challenging people's belief systems that they have devoted their careers and lives to serving can push them into a life crisis, and we who are carriers of change, of a new way, need to be aware that we will be caught in the administration's internal conflict between something that wants to open and something that doesn't." It is only through understanding these often encountered feelings and reactions that we can begin to engage in more dialogue and move into a more facilitative role around these conflicts. Conflict for me is a symptom of not knowing each other well enough, and it can often be a first step in getting to know each other better. A facilitated conflict often moves and new alliances are formed. As much as I felt that administrators often jumped to judge our work, I also jumped to judge their being so closed at times. The official reason for why I couldn't work was usually that classic double bind that says, "We really do want you to work here as soon as you can produce definitive quantitative data," the magical key to the world of the measurable. This was both the discussion in this hospital with this administrator I mentioned earlier who asked me to leave his hospital, and other hospital administrators, and is a discussion I have had with so many medical professionals. Then I would say, "I would love to produce such data, please help me to be able to work in your hospital so I can gather such data." The discussion often circled like this for quite a while. These days I am more open and say, "I understand your thinking, and your feeling cautious about change does have a point. You are open to data in a form that is comfortable for you. I would love to give you that data, and I also understand that you may already be at your limits by being open to receive the data, and at this point you may not feel open to helping me gather the data."

One of the chief administrators of a huge Israeli treatment center, whom I mentioned earlier, once told me that he was just too close to retirement to be open to such a radical change. I appreciated that so much more than his just throwing me out. A path of compassion and conflict resolution led me to pursue the relationship with him. I liked so much how he put his arm around me when we met. Also, there are rank issues involved. At the time I was seeing him only as this huge fig-ure with so much rank, and I forgot to see the human being who needed to be seen, recognized, appreciated, and respected. We were practicing what Pierre is referring to as relationship-style medicine with each other. We were being our real selves, meeting, being vulnerable and real, and in this context, healing can occur. I felt healed from his previously having thrown me out of his hospital so quickly. He told me how, at one point in his life, he had been like me, full of curiosity and hope and experimentation. He also told me some of what life was like for him now, as his personal and family life was entering a new phase. We met each other and could see the commonality. He didn't let me work there, but it was alright. Many other places let me in; he was a time spirit, a role, trying to hold back the gates of change, and the times were changing. He was representing the resistance to change, and change happened anyway.

Ten years later, I now understand much more about how challenging the work that we are bringing is for others. I know people want to do the best they can for their patients, and working with coma patients is such difficult work. It requires everyone, whether nurse, physical thera-pist, physician, or administrator, to be incredibly dedicated. And then we come in and start challenging a key part of their paradigm. As the above administrator told me, they only treat the body. Day after day, I saw patients who were receiving great physical care but were spending hour after hour with very little interaction. Many times I would be working with someone and word would get out that exciting changes were happening, and suddenly when I went into the hall to take a break, family member after family member would grab me and try to pull me in to see their loved ones—"Just for five minutes, please doctor." I can imagine if I were an administrator what a shock that would be to me. I might start to worry: What if we have been missing something for all these years that we can't provide? What about our facts and figures that say people don't come out past this point? What do we do with those maps that we know, that our data support, and that we have been following for so long? In a way it is as if we are saying that in Coma Work the basic paradigm needs to shift. Those of us who have read Thomas Kuhn's classic *The Structure of Scientific Revolutions*[8] know that paradigm shifts take time, and that these shifts are full of resistance.

I have been helped greatly by looking at my own paradigms that I have trouble shifting out of and that I hold onto with such ferocity as if I am hanging on so I don't fall into the abyss. I can also be like the administrators who don't want to look at new paradigms. For example, I love to do Aikido, that mystical, practical, martial art. Our teacher is always saying, "softer, go softer, it is so much stronger." The first couple of years I looked at him like he was crazy. Someone grabbed me with force, and I gave them back enough fight so that they would know better next time. It took so much practice and consciousness to risk being soft when attacked. In Aikido, we call this using our Ki, our energy, rather than our muscles. Many experiences later, I am opening up to the change. I can move some of these huge men with my softness and energy whom I would never be able to budge with all my muscle. Yet I expected these administrators and physicians to open up to the soft approach of Coma Work. I am soft on the fixed time tables of when people may recover and soft on the interventions. We follow the person's direction in coma, believing that they will show us the way to be most helpful and facilitative to them. Yet I now feel I was not soft enough with the administrators. I forgot at times to take care of their need to be appreciated, respected even more, and to shine themselves. I forgot to be soft when I met rigidity, and I met force with force. Part of this softening is first burning my wood, that is, taking the time and space to express somewhere my frustration and anger with the system and how I have been hurt by it. I can still feel a bit of wood-burning going on in my writing. I also support my clients and in the case of Coma Work, both the patient in coma and the families, to express both their appreciation and frustration with the limits of the system they are working in and with. I don't think I could have taken a softer approach to life without first having been a very angry, one-sided person, but everything changes, including my being only on my own side and the one-sidedness against Coma Work practices like ours.

These days I carry myself differently in hospitals; I am much more open to all sides. I have changed and so have they. Recently I was welcomed into three hospitals in Israel. One specialized in bringing in all kinds of alternative medicine. They were actually thrilled to have me there working with one of their soldiers. The paradigm *is* shifting as Coma Work comes in under the umbrella of complementary and alternative medicine. I am not there to make their work harder, but possibly easier. I know that working with coma patients can be frustrating and depressing but Process-oriented Coma Work can make the work more interesting and offers more hope than a purely materialistic, physical body-based method.

THE ISSUE OF HOPE

I am often warned by physicians to be sure not to give the family false hope. What is false hope, though? If methods tend to produce results that the physicians are not used to, then this hope may be grounded in my experience and is not false hope. Hope and depression fill the coma wards, just like hope and depression fill the streets in war zones. There is so much hopelessness, and yet hope flairs. Sometimes it is false hope and sometimes genuine. What I try to do is give families and staff realistic hope by saying this is what I can just about guarantee will come out of the work, which is that you will feel more connected to the coma patient and feel more easily able to relate to them and to each other. The rest is up to nature. This cautious statement still represents a hopeful perspective for the patients we work with who are often only given a 0 to 5 percent chance of recovery.

Process-oriented Coma Work is ready for a leap into the next step of recognition. We are being welcomed in more and more settings to work and to do research. The paradigm is shifting, person by person, hospital by hospital. Nurses, in particular, have frequently run up to me and said "keep going, we know what you are doing and we see the changes." At last it is being recognized that rather than being there to threaten anyone, I am adding awareness and a bit of sunlight into what has often been one of the darkest, most hopeless kinds of medical conditions, and we are only just beginning. We have so many tools that are working, and we have so much more research and development to do to make these methods increasingly useful to our clients and their families.

Chapter 10

Post-Coma Work

In Chapter 9, we explored some of the systemic issues that we may encounter as helpers and when we practice Coma Work. In this chapter, we will describe the limitations and challenges coma survivors, their families, and helpers face once they recover from coma or remote states of consciousness.

Pierre: In 1975, Marilyn Price Spivack's then-teenage daughter suffered a brain injury in a car accident. Exasperated with the lack of specialized services and resources, Marilyn founded the Brain Injury Association of America, which is now the foremost advocacy organization for Traumatic Brain Injury (TBI) survivors in the United States. For Spivack the limitations of current service provisions are still glaringly apparent. Many states do not have a single brain injury rehabilitation center, and of the states that do offer some level of TBI treatment, few actually provide enough assistance to acquire even the most basic level of specialized care. At rates that can exceed $1,000 a day for post-acute TBI rehabilitation, there aren't many American families that can afford a month's worth of treatment, much less the usually recommended minimum of 90 days.

How many people need this provision, or how many people have a traumatic brain injury in the United States? According to the Centers for Disease Control and Prevention, of the 1.4 million who sustain a TBI each year in the United States: 50,000 die; 235,000 are hospitalized; and 1.1 million are treated and released from an emergency department.[1] The

number of people with TBI who are not seen in an emergency department or who receive no care is unknown.

What are the consequences of a TBI? The Centers for Disease Control
and Prevention estimates that at least 5.3 million Americans currently
have a long-term or lifelong need for help with daily living as a result
of a TBI.[2] Because the brain is complex, every brain injury is different.
Brain injury affects the injured person's subjective well-being, their self-
confidence, independence, and life satisfaction, and it changes his or her
social integration and social role; it can also impede the person's ability
to self-manage behavior, which can lead to agitation or violence and
lower barriers to the abuse of alcohol and drugs; it leads to depression,
post-traumatic stress disorder (PTSD)[3] and other psychiatric disorders,
and to unemployment because of the loss of job skills. Brain injury
itself is a chronic disease with high morbidity and mortality. Brain
injury survivors often have life-long motor function problems, injury-
related medical issues such as epilepsy and chronic pain, and cognitive,
psychiatric, and behavioral issues.

Medical treatment for brain injuries from the Iraq war will cost the
government at least $14 billion over the next 20 years according to a
recent study by researchers at Harvard and Columbia.[4] Spivack, who
currently works with the brain injured population at Spaulding Rehabilitation Hospital in Boston, states:

The military is doing an extraordinary job in saving young soldiers and treating them through the acute rehabilitation phase. Now the government must
make a commitment to help them in their recovery, but where are the resources going to come from? As brain-injury professionals, we know that TBI services aren't available in many places across the country, and we are aware of
huge holes in the system. Frankly, I'm frustrated and angry about the government's refusal to give the TBI population the support it desperately needs.[5]

An evaluation of TBI programs and services conducted by the Institute of Medicine reads like a list of indictments. It concludes that "finding
needed services is, far too often, an overwhelming logistical, financial, and
psychological challenge . . . the quality and coordination of post-acute
TBI service systems remains inadequate."[6]

In my past and current work, I encounter many individuals who have
suffered a brain injury. Many professionals speak of a silent epidemic.
By this they mean that the problem is not being recognized or adequately
addressed by either society or medicine. Similarly, many brain injured
individuals feel unrecognized in their struggle. Often their impairments
and disabilities are not visible from the outside. They suffer from combined

physical, emotional, and cognitive difficulties that do not easily fit into classical psychiatric or medical categories. Many people suffer from chronic uncharacteristic headaches and other neurological symptoms that defy medical understanding and treatment. Others struggle with severe behavioral and emotional problems and end up in long-term psychiatric care without adequate specialized treatment.

Carlos is a young Hispanic man who suffered a severe brain injury following a diabetic coma. The injury left him disabled with the intellectual abilities of a 12-year-old. In a fight, he threatened his sister with a knife, which led to a psychiatric hospitalization, referral for counseling, and placement in an adult foster care home. I am supervising some of the members of a multidisciplinary team who are in charge of his outpatient treatment. The problems they face are innumerable. Carlos's insulin-dependent diabetes requires ongoing monitoring and supervision. He is not only unable to follow his dietary prescriptions, but he also engages in addictive eating binges of junk food. Through coaching of his foster care team and behavioral treatment plans, we are trying to contain his impulsive eating and other emotional outbursts. His ongoing need for combined intense medical and behavioral supervision and treatment exceeds what he can afford and the structural medical resources available to him.

Many brain injured people have to reinvent themselves and find a new place in society. Many lose their former jobs and their friends. They feel stigmatized by the social bias that values people from a perspective of productivity. This is reflected in statements from individual patients I saw in my practice such as:

- "When we lose the ability to 'do' things we used to do before the injury, we feel like we have lost who we were."
- "We are not brain injured but persons with a brain injury."
- "You are not what you 'do.'"
- "We are human beings, not human doings."

In my work with Chris (see Chapter 4), an important focus was on supporting him and helping him to adjust to inner- and outer-biased perceptions of worthlessness and inadequacy. His depression was in part a reaction to feeling overwhelmed by unrealistic expectations and confronting cognitive and physical limitations. The dreaming and essence work we did together comprised of rediscovering his sense of freedom, space, and unhindered playfulness. Bridging his current experiences with childhood memories allowed him to find some meaning in what was also a random and fateful accident.

As a young adult, Carl, another client, participated in several bar brawls and suffered a series of blows to his head that injured his brain. Now in his 60s, he recounts how his personality changed since from then on. He remembers having difficulties performing certain intellectual tasks. He adjusted by engaging in a musical career as a blues and jazz saxophone player. But lately he has started to experience impulsive feelings of sadness and anger. His aging brain is becoming less able to compensate for the "impairments," and they have become more apparent again. I am a musician, too, and Carl and I spend hours talking about his music and the experiences he has feeling the sounds and vibrations of his saxophone. I use his musical talent to explore his impulsivity and ask him to include the strong emotions in his improvisations. With the help of his creativity, he is able to develop new coping skills. Beyond coping and adjusting to his disability, Carl and I are working on embodying his soulful musical spirit and creativity. His early accident directed him to a path of music that has become his life force and spirit. Unfortunately his early fights also injured his jaw, and teeth and dental problems are now threatening to incapacitate his saxophone playing. Under the stress of losing his music he has become intermittently suicidal. With guided imagery, I am helping him explore his fantasy of death and am enabling him to get in touch with a lost spiritual experience that was close to his peak experiences in music.

Coma and brain injury rehabilitation is a huge societal problem, and we invest far too few resources into it to even begin to address the multiple problems that individuals and families face. Specialized rehabilitation care is very limited and not accessible to most people. Working with individuals is not sufficient; we also need to work with health care administrators and government officials, and there is a huge need for advocacy and policy change. Nevertheless, I hope that some of the skills described so far can help ease some of the processes that individuals and families go through.

LOOKING BACK AND MAKING SENSE AFTER COMING OUT OF COMA

Gary: Throughout this book, we are saying that comas are life-changing experiences meant to alter the flow of your everyday life. They are an attempt that those deepest parts of us are making to come forward to be seen and heard. It is preventive medicine to pick up the messages behind the coma so that they don't have to somehow recycle and repeat themselves. Currently, coma therapy rarely focuses on the meaning of comas; as a result many individuals have experienced comas, fully recovered, and yet have not consciously understood the message of their coma. These messages are so powerful that they tend to continue to present themselves to us in the form of accidents, illnesses, addictions, and they are especially likely to come to the foreground when we are close to death. Picking up these messages in a consciously relaxed way can therefore be incredibly valuable. One of my friends repeatedly got knocked unconscious. That unconscious state flirted with her. When she deliberately went deeply into it, she found that some major shift in consciousness was trying to happen, which would allow her to open up to the altered states that are flowing through her constantly. Like most people, she used to push these other nonconsensus reality states aside, and they would push back by "knocking her out"! When she started to go into these knocked-out places intentionally, the concussions and head injuries stopped.

There are three major ways for people to re-access the coma experience. The first method is to do the basic Coma Work exercise of pretending they are in a coma, and then the coma worker facilitates them through the various steps of connecting and working with all of the minimal signals present. It is common for people who have previously had comas to go more deeply into these pretend comas then people who haven't had them. When people go through and process these states, they almost always have insights into what the states are about. Often one or two people in coma seminars have been in comas in the past. The meanings they discover are not just intellectual ideas, but may often express themselves through wild movement, sound, relationship, and other channels of awareness. Many comas are near-death experiences, and most such experiences somehow put the person more in touch with their most basic, essence-level experience. I always remember one man I worked with who described himself as having been nonspiritual up to that point in his life when he went into coma. However, he also told me that as a young man, he had been trapped under a car and had an experience that it was God who had saved him and brought him help. The coma was a return to this previous numinous moment in his life. Many people have these profound God-like experiences when processing coma.

The second way I work with post-coma people is to go back and work with how they came to be in the coma initially, we go back to that first moment when the heart attack or stroke or head injury or whatever occurred. For example, with auto accident victims, we go back into the posture they remember or associate with that accident. Often very specific information comes out of going back, with awareness, into those very first moments. There are currently several interesting books written by people who themselves were in the field of neurology and other brain sciences who describe the awareness they had during the first moments of a major stroke. *My Stroke of Insight* by Jill Bolte Taylor[7] is one of the most popular books that describe a brain scientist's personal inner-experiences during her stroke. These early stroke experiences are of things such as time stopping and of completely entering into the present moment. These are not just random experiences but profound life-changing events. I have worked with many accident victims who have been in and come out of coma. I take them back to the posture they remember for two reasons. The first is that shock hangs around for a long time after we recover from trauma, and by going into the experience consciously with awareness, much of the shock dissolves itself. And secondly, people make many discoveries about the accident. Sometimes I invite them just to watch as I act out the accident. At other times, I have them go into the posture and process their experiences as the victim of that accident, and then I have them become the thing that caused the accident and have them pick up its power. One of my clients had a very severe accident when her car spun out of control. It was the spinning state that she needed to pick up; until then she had been living her life step-by-step, and she had been much too linear. Several of my clients have been able to pick up the power of what hit them. That can be a bigger process to work with. I knew someone who had once been hit by a truck in her car. I know she had done some work with this, but then much later in life, she was struck by a train and killed. These are central life processes and they may take us a lot of time and attention to process, before we can pick up all of our inner force rather than just having it directed at us. All that force that came at her may have been part of her own secondary power that she hadn't fully identified with. Here is a brief exercise (Exercise 10.1) to practice this concept of processing the accident.

Exercise 10.1
Processing an Accident

1. Recall a time you were in an accident.
2. Put in one hand the part of you that was in the accident and in the other hand what caused the accident, like the car that hit you.
3. What is the message behind the thing that caused the accident?
4. What is its energy like? How did you or how do you need some of that energy in your life that was most affected by being in the accident?
5. If that same force and object were to come at you now, what would you say to it? What has changed since the accident? And what still needs to move more in you so that the accident isn't needed again? Let your hands show through interacting with movement what the next steps are in your development.

A third method I use is to work more psychologically, asking the person about the central issues, edges, and stuck places that were present in their life at the time of the coma, and about the changes that have happened since. It might be that something that is already emerging in the coma person's life needs to deepen. For example, let's say I was the one who had been in a car accident and I had gone into a coma. I would have said that before the coma there was a very busy part of me, and since the coma I have discovered a person who likes smelling flowers. Then my work would be to find a way to get those two parts connected. One way I might do this is to center myself and then put these two parts in different hands and let the hands interact and work on this polarity. In Process Work, we have many different psychological methods for working with polarities—from role playing both roles and going back and forth and helping them interact with each other, to going into our own deepest selves and having the sides interact while we stay connected to our clearest essence, to having someone play out these polarities for us. For example, one of my patients who recovered completely said that before the coma he was a total party guy, and after the coma, he became someone who was really serious about life, achieving his goals, etc. I used to go into my center and let these sides interact through me and watch his feedback. I would say something like "I love playing around and going to wild parties, but this other part of me is very serious." Then I would show him how he needed a bit more sobriety in his wild side to tame some of those wild parties and hangovers, and a bit more fun and freedom in his career pursuing path. I would show him how I would flow back and forth between these polarities, and I let his feedback guide me as to the best way to do this.

POST-COMA RECOVERY

There have been many excellent books on the stages of recovery of coma from all the different related healing modalities, including speech therapy, physical therapy, and the whole field of rehabilitative medicine. Yet I have found very little on psychological interventions to help people process their comas and come back after head injuries, major strokes, and other causes of coma. Process-oriented methods of recovery after coma could be a book in itself, and yet it is important we at least begin this discussion here.

I have worked with people who have been in coma for just a few days and with one man who was in a minimally responsive state for 12 years. In terms of recovery, I have had people come back in very different ways—some come all the way back very quickly, some all the way to pre-coma functioning very slowly, others who have come back only par-tially, and some who did not come back at all. All of the methods that we use with the person in the coma are relevant when we work with them as they come back, and now that the verbal component is often also present, I can receive not only nonverbal but also verbal feedback and expression. People come out of coma differently, just as they behave differently in coma. Some come out quietly and just wake up. Others wake up feeling violent. One woman just smiled and was slightly disori-ented. Another man began to pound on the walls and scream. He was able to read history and do math problems, but he would also spend hours in fits of rage. Still another man couldn't stop laughing.

Of course we can look at all these causally as the effects of brain injury on parts of the brain that are associated with impulse control, and they take time to recover, as does the ability to speak, walk, and other basic functions. However, the Process Work view is that these behaviors are also meaningful and relate to the central core of who we are. If you are in rage, that isn't just your brain not quite functioning properly yet, it is also something that has always been there that is simply not being inhibited at this moment. That man's laughter was always there, maybe it was a part of himself he had tried to reach and only had access to through drinking or drugs before the coma. So if someone is raging, we might work with them to complete that rage in movement and sound. I would help them to find out what is behind that rage and where is it directed. Is it just power or is it related to having to deal with the agony of recovery or at a parent or the system taking care of them? Is that humor an edge to something, or something childlike, or something with the utter detachment of Buddha? We can explore and find out.

The degree to which people recover may have a great deal to do with effectively processing the event that led up to, and was responsible for, the coma. With the woman who came all the way back from having almost been murdered (see Chapter 5), I began to process all of that immediately. The first movement I could see that she really wanted to make was a punch to my hand. She made it repeatedly as she started to come out of coma. At each point we would process the violence that had happened to her. After she made a psychological breakthrough in terms of expressing her hurt and anger in movement, she would sud-denly be able to move her arms or her legs more, or her throat and speech would open up more. Mind and body together processed her feelings of moving from almost murder victim to powerful woman in charge of her life. Physical and speech therapy helped on the physical level, but more was needed than just physical healing. Her body was wracked with all kinds of trauma responses that needed to thaw out and express themselves fully. Once she did this, her body repeatedly made progress that had previously been considered anywhere from medically unlikely to medically impossible. On the other hand, clients who don't get the psychological follow up may not make as much progress. One man I worked with who had been given no chance of recovery spoke after just one day's work. We worked on his mind-body and we discussed the issues and circumstances that led to his coma. We also worked with his wife and family. We were working in another country, and after a short time we had to return home. He never spoke again, in spite of all the excellent physical care he was given. This whole area of mind-body in coma recovery needs a lot of research. My hypothesis is that there would be a dramatic change in the depth and speed of improvement in patients receiving on-going Process-oriented work.

SYMBOLIC THINKING AND THE PATH BACK

When words come back, they don't always make sense on a consensus reality level. The words mean something on a symbolic level similar to our dreams. To work with people recovering from coma, we need to be able to translate dream language just as if it were Spanish or French or Japanese. It *is* understandable; it just needs translation. In more mainstream rehabilitation practices, these words are often ignored or viewed as just crazy brain injury talk, but I have never yet experienced a case where the words meant nothing. Remember my earlier story (Chapter 5) about the man who recovered from stroke, whose speech wasn't considered by the medical staff to be meaningful or significant unless it was three logical sentences in a row?

My favorite example about discovering the meaning behind seemingly meaningless words is my client, Steve, whom I worked with in the southern part of the United States. Steve was recovering from a massive stroke. When he first started to talk, he had one favorite thing to do. He would sing the song "She'll be Coming Round the Mountain When She Comes." I would play with him with that song, and mostly what we did was emphasize the "*when she comes, when she comes*" part of the song. We would play with those words. I would sometimes take them further and say she will be coming round the mountain when she is good and ready, and he would then sing back "*when* she comes, *when* she comes," emphasizing the *when* part of it. We were all pushing Steve to get it together and come back for all of us. He was telling us something about his process, saying something like, "When nature is right then I will be back. I am following nature, not you." As he was recovering, Steve, who had sold things all his life, tried to sell me the things in his room—the drapes, the pictures, all very cheap, about five cents! As we worked with this, I began to get a sense he was telling me, "all these material trappings aren't where it's really at, Gary." He continued to recover, at his own pace, to his own level. His death was similar, having a quality of following his own timing. He is a teacher in that way to his family: don't get hung up on pushing things, and especially don't get caught up in materialism. As I knew the family, I could see not only the apparent randomness of his speech, but also the wisdom of his message. We could all meditate on that. Next time you are pushing a project or healing or making love, try following nature's timing, not just pushing to reach a goal. Next time you get overly materialistic, ask yourself if your things are really worth the price you are willing to pay for them.

I think back also to the young man who laughed so much. The staff would ask him all kinds of serious questions and he would laugh, tell jokes and be really silly. I am on the staff side first, if you want to go out in the world, you had better be serious and answer questions and only laugh at the proper times, and yet I am with my client also. If you've just made it back from the doorway of death and coma, how can you take all those things so seriously? Imagine if you had just found your way back from death and coma. You've put your brain back together so you can now walk and speak and think, and someone is asking you typical mental status questions (such as who is the President of the United States, or what year is it?). Can you imagine that you might also feel like laughing? It is like someone making it back who has been lost in the snow on the mountain and people keep asking them if they are upset they missed a few days of work. From the place of depth and detachment that the journey took you to, you can only laugh. At that moment, you don't get the consensus reality scene, and the consensus reality scene doesn't understand the world you have been to; in terms of timing with these patients, they come around the mountain when they come, and that they come back at all is often miraculous.

ROADBLOCKS

The challenge of coming out of any extreme state is that your life is still there when you come back, and part of the extreme state may have been to do with taking a break temporarily or hopefully permanently from that life. Part of the job of the coma worker is to help process that life situation so that it also changes. The coma changes the person, but then they have to face the same life circumstances again. Post-Coma Work for me has often involved individual, couple, and family therapy to deal with what is still there. In one situation, I worked with the woman, and with her children, and with the whole family, all to make adjustments to the reality of the post-coma person and to the situation before the coma. For example, the children needed to adjust to the fact that their mom was going to be much more clear and assertive than before the coma, as well as much more focused around her career. Again we have to address who this new person is, and then support them to transform their outer reality so that the outer reality doesn't force them back into the same situation that fed the coma situation.

CHANGING SOCIETY

My coma patients and I have a joint task. As they come out of comas, I am helping them not just to adjust to their families and society, but also to bring back their information and changes to their relationships, families, work, daily lives, spiritual paths, and society as a whole. This is the political part of Coma Work. If I just help them readjust, I may be undermining the whole work they have done for themselves in the comatose state and by getting out of it. Many of the patients I have worked with have been in Israel. Sometimes they are soldiers. Other times I have worked with those involved in suicide bombings and were caught in an explosion that put them into coma. These comas are happening right in the middle of the political turmoil of the world. I talk to the coma patients about the world, helping them to make meaning of their injuries and do something together to deal with the agony of war, or whatever may be part of the societal-based causes that are part of the picture of their coma. I remember challenging a woman caught in the middle of a suicide bombing to come out of the coma and do something about this mess that led to her coma. She responded when we worked, but unfortunately I was limited to only one day with her. There is no such thing as just an individual problem. Each problem has all the levels of individual, relationship, group or family, and world present. If I am working with a man whose wife says he had a stroke the first time she refused him sex, that coma is about him and his brain and his sexuality; his relationship with his wife; and also his culture, which is in transition around male and female issues of power, especially as they relate to sex. Coming back may mean facing and working with and becoming part of the changes happening, and not just feeling like a victim of these changes.

Paul is another good example. He wanted to be an artist and a lover, but his family wanted him to be a doctor or a lawyer or anything but an artist. His coming out of the coma is political, not only in his family but also in a culture that says art is nice as a hobby but it's not a real job. Coming out of the coma means facing the reality of that particular culture and transforming it. In Native American traditions, people go on vision quests. They might fast and sit on a mountain for a few days seeking a vision. The vision is not only for their personal life but also for their community. The medicine man or woman helped make sense of this vision quest for the individual and for the community as a whole. The Process-oriented coma worker sees their client as potentially on a vision quest. We are the shamans helping them to come back and make sense of their visions and to help them bring this vision into their community. One of my clients was invited to speak about her recovery after she came all the way back from the gate of death, following a violent attack. She also told me to talk with the newspapers and help a columnist to write about her journey and about our work together so that, together, we could teach something about courage, healing, and domestic violence. Part of her healing was to make this stand—to make her journey valuable to others.

So in summary, post-coma recovery is a lot like other parts of Coma Work. We work with the individual, with the people and family they are in relationship with, with the system the person is involved with in terms of their healing and recovery, and with the overall world that makes this world a tough place for so many to live in and to want to return to, once in coma. We help people to find their way back by following their process and help them to interact with and change the world they are coming back to.

Chapter 11

The Future of Coma Work

This chapter summarizes the work so far and suggests possible future developments. There is also a dialogue between the authors on the major issues covered by the book, their awareness of the cultural debate, and the possible and necessary directions for the future of this field. The hot issues they discuss include differing views of death and dying; how present and responsive the coma patient is; belief in the possibility of and timing of recovery; conflicting ideas about advanced directives and the ethics of the withdrawal of life support; and specifically the timing of the withdrawal of life-sustaining measures.

Gary: As the book is coming to an end, I notice I am having a debate with myself:

Gary, did you give them enough detail on how to do this work? Well, probably not, but there are other books that cover the basic details. I want to give the reader a sense of where this work is going and can go.

Well then, Gary, maybe you are spreading false hope. If I am, it is to counter all the hopelessness and depression around people in comas.

Still Gary, you may be spreading false hope. That is a valid point in that I should talk about more cases that I didn't feel very good about; however, I am standing for some kind of balancing of a system that tends to write off recovery very quickly and that measures progress only in big leaps and that views death as a failure.

OK, Gary, let's say you get through to people and people want more of this work. Are you and Pierre going to be able to do all that work yourselves?

Well, we can do some of it, and there are others besides the two of us with training and experience in this work. Actually, there are many people trained who just need and want more experience, so maybe this book will open up doors for them.

Gary, you still seem too one-sided toward recovery. Well, yes, I am still one-sided, but I am also much more open to viewing death as a success and to understanding that some people will not move at all no matter how much I work with them. Yet I don't want to give up my love and hope that people can come back from coma if it is right for their process.

Gary, you make it sound like it is some kind of conscious choice, and if people don't come back it is because they don't want to. Well, dear inner arguing voice, you have caught me again. Before I finish, I need to be clearer and say that what direction someone in coma goes is a matter of so many factors—physical, psychological, spiritual, family, and cultural. I am not saying at all that it is some kind of conscious choice to come back or not. In fact, I see part of our job as clarifying the issues and processes for the person so that they may begin to approach a point where they have some choice.

Gary you never discussed the money issues of Coma Work. OK, Voice, I thought we could get through this book without mentioning it, but I see we can't, so I will do it now. Partly I am reluctant to speak about it because the money is complicated. Someday hopefully this work will be covered by health insurance. We have worked with people who have needed Coma Work from one end of the spectrum who couldn't pay for my dinner if I worked for them, to people who could afford to have built us a whole hospital. We do our best to try to help everyone and to balance out those who can pay and those who can't.

OK, but then how can you charge regular rates for something you can't guarantee? Well dear voice, there are very few guarantees in medicine or in psychology. The ethical thing for me is to tell people exactly what to expect and what not to expect. I try to be as transparent as possible, and then I let them make their own choices.

Thank you dear inner arguer, I appreciate that all the points you are bringing up are helping me bring this discussion right down-to-earth. We have had chapters where we talk of spirituality, of miracles, of different levels of consciousness, and that leads me to think about what I really want people to take from this book. First and foremost, I want people to see that this form of psychology belongs in Coma Work. It is not just up to medical doctors and nurses and physical and occupational and speech therapists to do what they can for the physical body. They do a great job, but the person's chances of having a more positive experience are greatly enhanced through the addition of psychological work. I want professionals as well as families of loved ones to understand this and utilize this work.

I want people to know that we understand to a great degree why this work is effective, and we also know that working with states like this are full of mystery. I want people to understand that this kind of work often brings significant positive changes in a loved one, but it is certainly no guarantee. We often work with people who have been given less than 5 percent chance of recovery, and those are tough odds to work with. I myself will be happy if this book causes families and professional caregivers to integrate any of this approach, even if it is just realizing that the person is somehow present, and that what they are doing in coma is somehow meaningful to their evolution.

Since I began doing Coma Work, I have seen slow but steady shifts toward two main trends. The first is the deepening of this work as Process-oriented Psychology deepens. Drs. Arnold and Amy Mindell have continued to lead the evolution of this work into the realm of sentience and essence work, which the Mindells call the second training. The first training is more signal-oriented and is what Coma Work was originally based on. Through our theory and stories, we have been illustrating how we work with both the first and second training in this work. We are not only working with signals that can be seen, but with our deepest intuitions, and we are and bringing in our own feeling information and relating to our clients in this way. Our work includes both signal work and more intuitive work. But most essentially we follow the clients' feedback, which may come in the form of direct positive sensory-grounded signals from the client or as synchronous signals from the environment.

As I have become more and more connected with my own essence, my style of Coma Work has changed, as I discussed particularly in Chapter 8, "Coma as Teacher." The deepening of the work helps me to follow nature more closely and to be less easily polarized into a position of helping get the patient out of the coma state and back to normal. I am moving from the role of a healer to that of a facilitator of process, in whatever direction that river flows. I understand why we tend toward pushing and trying to bring people out of their comas. Not only do the families push, but also having a new method that was so marginalized by the medical systems we were working with resulted in my feeling that I had something to prove. As I learn from my patients and grow along with them, I am relaxing and being more present with them and the work.

The second trend I am aware of is that some of the problems with the medical system are changing. With the development of the new technologies, recent medical research is beginning to verify what we have been saying is happening, for example, about the potential for the development of new neural pathways. Pierre has talked about some of these ideas earlier, and it seems that each new technological development helps to verify the directions our Coma Work is going.

Another way I view this development is that Process-oriented Coma Work is like a nighttime dream that is manifesting. Our night dreams sometimes help prepare us for coming changes—changes that are, in fact, already happening but which our conscious mind is not yet picking up. As Process-oriented coma workers, we have helped prepare the field, so that now that what we have been talking about can be seen on a PET scan, it is easier to accept and make changes based on that new information. Part of what Coma Work has taught me is about how to help facilitate change in the theory and practice of scientific methods. I am more patient now, understanding from the inside and outside of our resistance; I see change happening in the moment as it arises in many small ways one patient, one family, one physician, and one hospital at a time.

Coma Work can benefit such a wide variety of people, including patients and their families, the caregivers including Process coma workers, and the general public. In a society that so strongly emphasizes being extroverted and verbal, Coma Work teaches all of us, coma patients and all the rest of us, how to be more internal and to process these deep inner states. Many of us could also benefit from learning to follow nonverbal signals more. I am still shocked when in my regular therapy practice I hear couples who have been together for 25 years say that they had no idea that their partners didn't like being touched intimately the way they had been touching them. Whether a lover or a dentist, an accountant or a friend, we all know what it feels like when we are with someone who can really follow and flow with our feedback. They are more relaxed and we are also more relaxed in their presence. Coma Work offers inner work and nonverbal communication and feedback skills for all who need them.

Meditation, sex, yoga, drugs, alcohol, dancing, athletics, all of these alter our states and tend to bring us out of our consensus reality minds and into deeper parts of ourselves. In a culture that tends to marginalize so many of our inner experiences, we need all of these ways and more. Coma is another way of altering our states. I am convinced that if more of us had easier access to the methods we are presenting in this book, we might be less likely to go into coma; if we did go in, we would have an easier time going through this doorway of comatose experiences. In Phillip Kapleau's *Wheel of Life and Death*, he talks of Zen Master Ikkyu on his deathbed. He said, "I shan't die, I shan't go anywhere, I'll be here. But don't ask me anything, I shan't answer."[1]

I want to say thank you, dear coma patients, for being our Zen masters and teaching us that being present is the eternal now; you are very present and we can join you in presence, even if it isn't the kind of presence we are comfortable with or used to. You are present, you just don't answer in normal ways, and in your not answering, we must open up and hear and feel and perceive in ways that go beyond our known ways, and in that way, together we are learning to be free from the limits of the unknown and to go together into the mystery.

Many of us feel uncomfortable with how different you (the coma patient) are in communication and in your states of consciousness, but I want you to know that it isn't just your work to come out and meet us. Together we must find a common ground where we can dance together and weave together our states of consciousness. For you, we may be a bridge back to ordinary reality, and for us, you are often a doorway into the unknown. May we continue to help each other grow, and may we as a society pick up all of the states of consciousness that you bring forward. We hope by doing that we will lighten your load.

Again I thought I had finished but here comes my internal figure with more challenges for me.

Gary, you thought you were finished, but I caught you trying to escape a few points. Well, go figure; do we have to do it all in one book?

No, Gary, I don't, but you need to go further here. You addressed the world issues a little bit, and you spoke about how the coma person reflects those world issues. I understand you are presenting them as part of the shadow of society, which needs to be integrated. You even mentioned above how, as a society, we need more relationship to this state of withdrawn consciousness as well as to our state of ordinary consciousness. Good so far. But you haven't said anything about how we are all in a coma. You need to explain how the coma person is not only reflecting the family system they are in, but also the world. Oh, dear inner figure, you've caught me again. I was hoping to skip this, but now that you press me, I must say something. For me, the world is in a coma in so many different ways. We are slowly waking up to some core issues such as racism, sexism, classism, environmental issues, economic disparity, hunger, poverty, and so many other issues. However, there is still one aspect where collectively we seem to stay in coma, and that is our international pattern of choosing war as our primary method of working with conflict. That process itself is like working with a coma, and that aspect of consciousness is so way down and locked in that I am not sure how to even begin to bring it out.

Well Gary, if as you say your methods really work and are holographic, then what has been working with the coma patients should also teach you about working with the world; therefore, you already know quite a bit about helping stuck states everywhere, including the world. Ah, thanks inner challenger, for holding me to that. What I have learned from Coma Work especially is to give all parts space and time, and to facilitate between the parts. This also is my hope for the comatose state I call war. I am hopeful that if I don't just go against this state and if I also help those who are interested in war to explore what is behind that state and help them to interact with the pro-peace people, something positive might really happen. I see this in the work I do in the Middle East. If I can create the same kind of space I create when working with coma patients, then people on all sides, for example, in the Israeli-Palestinian conflict, can begin to wake up out of the frozen, coma-like state. Then all kinds of things start to slowly move. For example, moments of processing trauma happen rather than just being frozen in trauma. The frozenness of hopelessness comes forward and begins to wake up some hope out of coma. In Coma Work, we learn the paradox of acceptance. Instead of forcing someone awake, we sit with the comatose states and unfold the meaning and presence in these states.

In war zones, I am learning the same lessons. If I just declare war on war, and I am always in conflict with conflict, then I keep the state frozen. Without facilitation, these sides remain in their frozen, polarized places forever. If I take one side or the other, I help to keep it frozen, just like if I take one side or the other and perpetuate polarization, I help keep the person frozen in coma. The problem is that whichever side I am on from my frozen state, I stop caring about the other side. If, for example, I just support the part of the person in coma who doesn't want to come back, and support them to stay in coma, I may just be supporting a side that may be suicidal, homicidal, hopeless, waiting for someone to pull the plug for their life to end. However, this may marginalize the part that wants to come back if life could be different and believes change is possible. If I can embrace conflict and recognize that I myself am as full of conflict as the outside person in coma, or the outside war scene, then at that moment I can begin to get interested and work on this, and my being facilitative may be very helpful. I have discovered that one of the most important feeling attitudes I can bring forward, or as Amy Mindell calls these skills meta skills, is curiosity. I bring a curiosity and am as open-minded as I can be, turning over rocks and asking what is under this rock? I find all kinds of stories, histories, and ghosts under the rocks, just like I find when I turn over some stones in the coma person's life. Without facilitation, war zones become fields of hopelessness, no one is able to be the curious mind that asks how did we get here, and how do we move on from here? The war zones are just like the coma wards where the action continues but no one is really checking in with what is happening. Both are just unfacilitated extreme states. For short periods of time both can seem relieving. Going consciously unconscious, pretending you are in a coma for an hour or so, can be a real joy. At first, war can seem ecstatic. I remember the excitement when the Iraq war began. People kept watching these amazing missiles on television that looked like giant fireworks, and how they were going to easily win us this war and save us. Being in a coma for months, or watching the Iraq war as people become physically and psychologically injured and the dead bodies come home, is a whole different experience. It wakes us up. What were we doing when we went unconscious and became so excited in the first place? For some people I am sure it is like that in coma. They went in needing this space so much, but now they just want to get back out of there somehow. They have had enough.

It is, however, not easy to accept any kind of symptomatic state; our tendency is usually just to go against it. Last week, I had the flu for two days. Two days of the flu is not so bad. However, I had to leave and teach in Canada, and I was worried I wouldn't be well enough to leave and teach. I worked for a few days on embracing the flu state. I was so against it. It was just what I needed. It took me down into my body, into rest, into the Earth, and into incredible dreaming realms. I found a dream figure who was a shaman who could glide across sand. He has a kind of slow, deep presence. It turns out this was exactly what I needed in this seminar. One of the participants at the workshop asked me to slow down this time and not cover as much ground but to go deeper and slower. I did, and got really good feedback. Even so, I had to work and work to accept this figure and to get it and the speedy, achieving, often driven part of me to relate to each other. As soon as I did, the flu seemed to go away quickly and completely. No wonder it is so much harder for us to not go to war against this comatose figure that seems so different than us. It is easy to become demanding: What are you doing in there for so long? Why don't you do more? Why don't you get better like most of our patients? Don't you know you can be depressing for us as doctors and nurses and therapists? We work so hard and you change so little. You become our least favorite patients, sometimes, even though we don't want to admit it. You remind us of parts of ourselves and our world that doesn't want to or can't change quickly. How can I believe that you are somehow part of this person's development? I can't even easily accept that two days of the flu might be a useful course adjustment and be meaningful for me.

So this is the work. We work with the paradox that if we first accept certain states as meaningful, that then permits change to occur if it wants to happen. Otherwise, I am like the person trying to unfreeze the frozen river by dumping my own bags of ice on the river. One of the first things I say to a person in coma, I could also say to the people when I work in war zones, or when I get the flu, or when I stop believing in my primary relationships. Ah, those magic words. Dear client, dear relationship, dear reader, dear world, believe in what is happening, believe in your experience. Breathe into it, and follow what is happening with your awareness and I will follow you. In Process Work, we reaffirm the deep wisdom of our beings and the wisdom beneath that organizes all things. We reaffirm our belief in Process Mind that arises out of our experience, when we can stay very close to the moment-to-moment unfolding of our process, as the river starts to flow again, and as that flow gains momentum. That momentum can bring us out of coma, can free us to live or die, can throw us into the arms of our enemies with a hug rather than a gun. This is the hope I want to convey in this book.

And here comes that inner debater again.

OK, Gary, for the moment I am satisfied. This last part touches me. It is what I was looking for before moving on. I do hope that Pierre and you will touch on some of these points in dialogue before ending, but for the moment I am satisfied. Dear critic, we appreciate you bringing up so many issues of group process, and we want to raise some further questions, knowing that we in this context can only answer them briefly. These are tremendously important issues and each one would each take many chapters to address fully, but our intention here is to give you, dear reader, a little more to think about, and to stimulate your thinking and dialogue and further group process. These questions cannot be answered by one or two people or experts alone, but are discussions that challenge us to get together and examine and define our values and our direction and our solutions.

Question: What is unique about Coma Work? How does it differ from medical approaches and other coma stimulation methods?

Gary: In terms of medical approaches, this is rather obvious. Medicine focuses on the physical body. Coma Work focuses on the physical body and the Dreambody, which involve the physical, emotional, and spiritual aspects of the person. We work with what is right in front of us, which is local to the person, and with the field around them, which is non-local. Medicine and most other Coma Work approaches follow a program where the goal is to get the person better. Process-oriented Coma Work follows the person and their unique process. The goal is increased awareness, wherever this leads the person. This belief in trusting and following awareness as the goal makes this approach unique.

Question: What are the minimal skills you recommend for someone who doesn't have much time to get trained?

Gary: Minimal training would be to know how to do the basic steps of Coma Work and to know something about how to work in each of the main channels of experience the patient might be in. You should also know about following the verbal and nonverbal feedback of both the client and their family.

Question: Why are you spending so much time and energy with people with such little chance of recovery? Is it ethical to bring someone out who may only come partially back? What are your ethics? How do you know they wouldn't rather be in a coma or dead if they can't be "normal and their old self"?

Gary: My main ethic is to do no harm, and this means I am careful and stay aware in my work to bring about further well-being in the client. Secondly, my deepest ethic is to follow the person's process. Sometimes it is difficult to determine the direction of their process and I must ask many times, especially, for example, if I am trying to get binary feedback on whether or not the client wants to die. I believe in a multi-state ethic and that my job is to help clarify the client's feedback on many issues and to guide the family toward an ethic, which says that big decisions need to come from more than just one part of a person's psychology. We want to get confirmation from several different states of consciousness. We usually refer to this as a two-state ethic, and sometimes this moves beyond two states to three or more states of consciousness, including waking and consensus reality, dreaming, and essence states of consciousness.

Pierre: Thank you, Gary, these are great and important questions. My first ethic is also to do no harm. Then after that, it is about doing my best to follow and respect the person's Process, both individually and in his or her family and social context. When should we hold ourselves back from intervening in our patients' natural processes? How do we know that we are following their wishes? In the Appendix, we refer to living wills and coma or remote state directives. These advance directives are documents that patients create to express their treatment wishes in the event that they are unable to respond and express what they want from their caregivers and helpers. These directives assume that our opinion about what we want is static and won't change once we are in a different state of consciousness. A longer term comatose or unresponsive state appears scary from a consensus reality and healthy vantage point. Typically, people who sign advance directives state that if they go into a coma or a vegetative state and there is no hope for a meaningful recovery, then they would want their caregivers to abstain from using any life-sustaining measures. It seems natural that we want to avoid being left in such a state. On the other hand, we don't know what our experience will be once we are in such a state. In such a state, we might have very different feelings.[2] From the outside, the experience may seem meaningless, but it may not be once we are actually experiencing it. Because of this dilemma we have developed the concept of a dual-state ethics or two state ethics. The dual-state ethics reflect an intention to assess a person's wishes from his or her previously written directives or known wishes as well as from their momentary remote, comatose, or unresponsive state. Information from both states is essential to make a decision. The question is: How do we accurately assess someone's wishes if they can't respond or communicate verbally? This is obviously very difficult and may not always be possible. But our belief is that we should at least try using our Coma Work skills such as sensitive body-oriented and binary communication techniques. When you think that up to 40 percent of the patients who we assume to be in a vegetative state are actually fully conscious but unable to communicate,[3] then the dual-state approach seems very relevant. For example, Chris, whose story I told in Chapter 4, is not his normal old self. Fortunately he wasn't in a situation in which the withdrawal of life sustaining measures was a possibility. But it could easily have been the case. Chris is struggling with significant cognitive and physical consequences following his accident; he probably will be on lifelong disability measures. But he is very resilient and able to learn to make sense of his new situation and self.

Question: What do you consider success and positive outcome, and why do some people come back from coma and others don't?

Gary: This is one of the great mysteries of the universe: when we live, when and why we die, and when and if and why we heal. My own experience suggests that the greatest possibility for someone to come back is if we can follow their Process openly and accurately, supporting who they are in the coma, and helping them to work on the unfacilitated conflicts present in their coma. We can help them work these issues out and ease their path back into waking life, and this gives people an incredible opportunity. Whether or not they recover depends, among other things, on their medical condition before and during the coma; their general interest and desire to come back to ordinary consciousness; their powers and abilities to make the journey; and last but not least, the skills of the coma worker.

Pierre: Predictions about coma recovery are very difficult to make. In my experience we have seen patients recover whose brain scans showed huge physical traumas and other patients remain unconscious who had minimal visible damage to their brain. In general, allopathic medicine considers that people who experience brain damage due to lack of oxygen (when the brain receives insufficient oxygen because the heart is not working efficiently) have a poorer prognosis than people who experience a brain injury from an accident. In addition, panels of medical experts have published guidelines stating that someone who remains in a vegetative state for more than three to six months after hypoxic brain injury and more than one year after TBI has very little chance of making a meaningful recovery. These prognostic predictions are based on consensus reality experiences and they disavow other experiences. They are also based on the current state of medical knowledge that is still very limited. We really don't understand coma and consciousness enough to make any sensible predictions. The concept of positive outcome also implies that coma and vegetative states are negative and not meaningful. This might be true from a consensus reality perspective. Of course they are painful on many levels: possibly for the individuals, certainly for the families and for the communities who carry much of the cost burden, etc. On another level, coma is one of nature's processes. In many places and for many years, people just died. In places with advanced medical infrastructure, people are now kept alive for much longer and some have the opportunity to regain cognitive abilities and physical functions. I think we have no other choice than to expand our understanding of these liminal states. Now that we have the technical knowledge to keep someone alive, we have to learn more about these non-ordinary states of consciousness and how to communicate with people who are in them.

Gary: Success for me consists of two main aspects. First, for the individual we are working with, success would mean that that person has more awareness of who they are and what is happening to them, and more access to making conscious decisions about their next steps. For the family, success means increasing communication with their loved one who is in a coma.

Question: As a skeptic and critical thinker, I wonder if you are just following your own beliefs and projecting onto the client; how do you know you are really connecting with them and their development?

Gary: This is very complicated, because there are more divisions than those stated in the question. For me, I can tell when I am projecting what I think should happen because it is reflected back in the feedback of the client. If my direction isn't the client's direction, it quickly becomes obvious. Coma patients don't have to adapt to consensus reality, so I can only push them so far in my direction and against their direction before I am frozen out with negative feedback. However, this question misses something entirely, which is that there is a place where it is all true—where, yes, I am projecting something onto the client, but the client and I are entangled, by which I mean that our growth is deeply connected. Our surface lives may be very different. The client in coma and I out of coma look and act very differently, but we may be sharing very similar directions and working on similar issues in our lives. Interventions which come from this place of entanglement will feel very different to the coma worker, and will engender very different kinds of positive feedback.

Pierre: This is again a great and also complex question. Rom Houben's story elicited a lot of public debate and controversy.[4] Some scientists said Rom's answers weren't really his answers, but actually that the helpers projected answers and they accused the helpers of having used facilitated communication. Facilitated communication is a process that was developed by some therapists who worked with severely autistic children. In this communication process the therapists support the hand or arm of a communicatively impaired individual while using a keyboard or other device with the aim of helping the individual to develop pointing skills and to communicate. The procedure is controversial, because a majority of scientific studies conclude that the typed language output attributed to the clients is directed or systematically determined by the therapists who provided the facilitated assistance. So it is really important to question yourself and wonder whether or not you are projecting your own hopeful expectations. One way of avoiding this problem is to include the whole care team in assessing someone's progress and responses. Helpers will have individual results from interacting with someone in a comatose state. Comatose people react differently to different individuals; they may "dislike" a certain helper and be more open to someone else. In Cenan's case (see Chapter 4), the family got much more of a response than the professional helpers. Working as a team allows us to be more differentiated. Comatose people also have times when they are more responsive. Any physical activity is a big strain for them which means that they need a break between interventions. If you don't get much response at a certain time, come back later and try again.

Question: Is the work different when someone is in coma because of a brain injury or a metabolic disease?

Gary: Yes, there is much more work to do putting the whole brain back together to come out of coma when someone has a brain injury, and the whole recovery period is much different. I will defer to Pierre on this question because of all of the medical differences involved.

Pierre: Gary is right. Metabolic changes from diabetes, renal failure, or liver failure can result in coma. These comatose states are often more fluid, especially when you correct the metabolic problem. When there is no structural damage to the brain, people can move in and out of coma very quickly. Of course, metabolic changes can over time lead to structural brain damage, too. You also often observe this fluidity of consciousness states at the end of life. The journey toward death—if death is really the process[5]—has many turns and ups and downs. Using Coma Work skills allows you to facilitate that journey and hopefully make it more meaningful.

Question: Do these methods of helping families make end-of-life care decisions up for the task? Are they reliable and exact enough for such weighty life-and-death decisions?

Pierre: In my opinion no one method by itself is helpful for big decisions. And no method is applicable without considering the context and feedback of the people involved. Advance directives are important, medical assessments are, too, and in addition, you can use binary communication methods to get the opinion of the person in the remote state of consciousness or coma. I also pay attention to non-local events. Suddenly a window or door opens, or a light goes on or off. Extraordinary things like this often happen around death and dying. It is also important that we allow ourselves to connect with our own dreaming and wait for answers to come. Working with someone in coma requires patience and openness to many types of responses from the person in coma. If you interact, wait for feedback. If there is a reaction, go on with what you are doing. In Coma Work, we use our own experiences as part of the Process. We are needed as we are! But how do we know if we are wanted or not? In my experience, comatose people's feedback is very sensitive. If they don't like what you are doing or if they need a break, they will withdraw. If they are with you, there may be a time delay before they react to you but they are there with you. For big decisions to happen, go slowly; repeat the questions at various different times and include everybody in the decision-making process and follow the group's feedback, too.

Gary: I think the biggest thing we can do to start being helpful is to give information. Often families are pressed to make these big decisions very quickly after their loved has gone into coma. I help them slow down and let them know that it often takes months to see what direction someone will go when they are in a coma. They don't have to make this decision on day three. I help families look at the situation with the most realistic eyes, neither overly biased by depression and fear nor by hope and illusion. I help families to ask the person in coma what they want to do about living and dying and to show this clearly. Finally, I help families understand that death is natural and a part of life rather than the failure of loved ones or of the medical system. I help them with their guilt and anger and grief and to process other difficult decisions so that the loved ones can make their decision from a clear place. I help them to look at medical prognoses, Process Work prognoses, and also their own dreams and intuitions to help them understand that a decision like this is full of feeling and relationship and to help them know that many shamans teach that to be a healer, we need not only to be able to help people heal and to come back to life, but also, when the time is right, to we need support their dying process, too.

Question: How is this work applicable with people who have dementia and are in the process of dying?

Pierre: With aging and at the end of life, people may go through changes that include non-ordinary states of consciousness. Memory loss, confusion, dementia, delusions, suspicions, agitation, and coma are some of the processes we can encounter in the care of the elderly. Coma Work skills can be very useful in helping people to navigate these transitional stages. In general there are no rigid steps and measures and no fixed rules in working with people. In my view, everything is a process; my methods and approaches depend on the context, the care team, their belief systems, and their feedback. Something that challenges many helpers is that clients near death often get agitated and try to get out of their beds. They might have visions of flying, going on a ship, riding on horses, falling into empty space, or going about their everyday life. A friend of ours on her death bed saw herself flying off as a mallard. Another friend faced the ocean as a golden tree and marched forward. Helpful methods are to join them and work with their visions and fantasies; help them choreograph, "fly" and "walk" with them, move their legs to help them get a sense of walking and flying, ask them to imagine where they are going and what they are doing, and follow their imaginary journey. This approach can reduce the agitation significantly. As a friend, family member, or caregiver, it helps you connect with the dying person's ultimate journey and will ease your grieving.

Gary: Yes, I agree. Our work is highly applicable to people with dementia and close to death in several main ways. First, our basic beliefs in following the Process, encouraging the people to believe in themselves, and valuing all states of consciousness including consensus reality, altered and dreamlike states, and essence states—all of these principles apply. We view the dementia not just as a deterioration of the brain but also as something that has meaning in the overall life flow of the person. In dementia states, for example, often something is erasing parts of the brain function, and while the eraser may be needed, it is often happening unconsciously. How can we help this person use the eraser part consciously? This is the same step we take in Coma Work. We look at what states come forward with the dementia, just like with the coma, and we ask ourselves: Is that some more primary state coming forward, or did the dementia or coma state knock out aspects of the primary process so something much more secondary could come forward? Often, because working with people with dementia means working in the verbal channel, we use the same skills we utilize when we are helping people recover from head injury, stroke, and other similar conditions. Words are used but not in such a consensus, logical structure, and we need to learn how to work more symbolically with the words as well as with their content. In terms of near-death and dying states, I use the same approaches all the time. Often near-death people are in and out of coma and other withdrawn states. One difference is, of course, that with someone I am helping over the last gate of death, I am emphasizing that direction, as opposed to coming back to life or helping to make a decision, as I am with the coma person. Still, I am working with the altered states in many different channels; working with the family system; addressing the attitudes and relationships with the hospital or hospice system—all these elements are there. We still view every moment, right up to the last moment of death, and probably beyond, as meaningful, as full of attempts to know ourselves, each other, and the universe. I have written more about this in my book, *Leap into Living*. One of the key short points to make here though, as Arnold Mindell has often said, is how frequently right before death people talk about going back to college. Just before my father died, he told Arnold that he wanted to come to Oregon to learn Process-oriented Psychology. So we keep helping the person grow and learn right up to that last second, and I find this greatly eases the dying process for the person who is dying and for everyone around them.

Question: Do you have a vision of where this work could go, or is your only goal to be useful to coma patients and help them slowly recover?

Pierre: My vision is for all of us to open ourselves up to learn from people who go through these states. In my view, they are teachers as are the families and caregiver teams. Coma Work is a co-learning process.

Coma is not just a pathological state that we need to fight; it is a meaningful experience for all of us. It comes with a lot of challenges and pain and it is inspiring. It touches on big questions of spirituality, and your beliefs about life and death. For us as communities and a society, coma presents a learning opportunity. Comatose people may help us revisit our ordinary everyday view of life. They help us get in touch with other levels of our lived experiences.

Gary: I see three major directions in Coma Work. The first one I see is that we are deepening and developing many more approaches to working with comatose states. Process-oriented Psychology is always developing new theory, depth, and approaches, and all of these changes need to be integrated into the Coma Work. Then we need to take this material and train coma workers, hospice workers, physicians, nurses, and family members of those who are in coma, and whomever else wants to learn. Second, we need more research to back up the effectiveness of what we are doing. Third, we need hospitals and nursing homes to welcome us in and to make this more of a part of the regular, ongoing treatment of coma patients. My congratulations go especially to my Process Work colleagues in Poland, who are now working closely with a new hospital being built in Warsaw specially to treat young people in comas, where Process Work will play a central role in the coma and family therapy work that happens there. I would like to see hospitals all over the world incorporate these methods.

Question: You both say in a way that the person in coma is a city shadow,[6] and therefore, the whole culture needs to make changes in its relationship to consciousness. How are you going to address the cultural issues related to coma beyond the individual, family, caregivers, and institutions you are directly involved with?

Pierre: I hope this book is a beginning and that it will be an inspiration for ourselves and others to take this work further.

Appendix

Glossary and Expanded Definitions

In this Appendix, we expand on some of the scientific and philosophical concepts developed in this book and provide some definitions of the medical and Process Work terms we have used. It will allow interested readers to delve deeper into some topics and to find helpful references and links.

Allopathy and Allopathic Medicine: Terms first described by Samuel Hahnemann, the founder of homeopathy. They are derived from the Greek words *allos* (other or different) and *pathos* (suffering). Allopathy means "other than the disease," and Hahneman intended to point out how, in contrast to homeopathic doctors, traditional doctors used methods that had nothing to do with the symptoms created by the disease. Both terms are now used to describe standard or traditional medicine.

Altered States and Extreme States: Process Work differentiates between altered and extreme states. These descriptions of mind states are nonpathological. Altered implies that your mind state differs from your ordinary state of mind. It ranges on a continuum from slight tiredness or foggyness through dreamlike states up to delusional and hallucinatory states. If the person's ability to relate the particular altered states to his or her ordinary state of mind is impeded and the person is overwhelmed by the state, then Process Work calls them extreme states. These states can be induced by mind-altering drugs, aging, fever, and other illnesses, as well as psychiatric conditions.

Anoxic Brain Injury: This occurs in cases of severe lack of oxygen to the brain. This usually happens when blood is unable to flow to the brain due to certain injuries or bleeding. There are three types of such injury: (1) blood does not carry enough oxygen; (2) toxins prevent oxygen in the blood from being used; and (3) no oxygen is being supplied to the brain, for example, because the heart is not pumping enough blood to the brain. The brain needs both oxygen and glucose to function properly. Brain cells begin to die after approximately four minutes without oxygen.

Archetype: Carl Jung used this term to suggest the existence of universal patterns that channel experiences and emotions, resulting in recognizable and typical behaviors. Mindell in his book, *The Dreamaker's Apprentice*, says, "Jung felt there were archetypes that created thematic patterns or blueprints that cultures used in their stories."[1] These archetypes are also present in and shape our individual dreams.

Authorization and Release/Informed Consent/Professional Disclosure Statement: We recommend that before you start practicing some of the methods described in this book with someone in coma, you should get an authorization and release from the patient's legal representative to do so. There are various ways to do this. Forms that are usually used in counseling and behavioral health are called Authorization to Release Information, Informed Consent, or Professional Disclosure Statement forms. Please ask your local legal and licensing authorities for the appropriate forms in your state and country.

Awareness: Awareness of the self and environment from a medical viewpoint depends on intact integrative neural connections between modular brain networks. These modules are relevant within the associative areas of the brain, which are all the expanses of the outer layers of the brain that have no specific sensory or motor functions, but instead are associated with advanced stages of sensory information processing, multisensory integration, or sensorimotor integration. Other brain networks that are relevant for awareness are connections between the association areas of the brain and the reticular formation for attention and wakefulness, the thalamus for synchronization, the hippocampus for cognitive memory, and the amygdala for emotional memory. These modular networks synchronize their state of excitement and form coherent meaning units, which can change in very short intervals.

Beliefs and Their Role in the Body's Physiology: Current medical understandings of how our beliefs are translated into our physiology are based on findings from mind-body medicine and our knowledge of the functioning of the human mind. Neurons are the fundamental cellular communication unit of the nervous system. Neurons communicate with each other by producing chemical substances called neurotransmitters that are sent across the synapses between neurons.[2] The action of these neurotransmitters (for example, serotonin) is the basis for brain functioning. These chemicals have been linked to behaviors as diverse as learning and memory, motor activity, thirst, pain, thermoregulation, pleasure, stress, emotions, mood, and sexual receptivity.

In addition, life course factors also interact with our contemporary circumstances both on a moment-by-moment basis and over time. The systematic differences in the quality of our environments and life paths shape the sculpting and neurochemistry of our central nervous systems. Animal studies have shown that their immune systems can be conditioned by outer events. Ader and Cohen[3] convincingly demonstrated that how we feel about the world can directly influence the competence of our immune systems. Moreover, the observation that the immune system can be conditioned implies that these effects can endure beyond the precipitating event. Thus, the nervous system that interprets the environment can also influence the long-term functions of the immune, hormonal, and blood clotting systems.

The two main organ sites for this "biological embedding"[4] of human experience are the autonomic nervous system and the hypothalamic-pituitary-adrenal axis (HPA). Together they mediate our adaptive response to stress by first initiating an increase in circulating catecholamines (for example, adrenaline or epinephrine) and glucocorticoids (such as cortisol) that alter the structure and function of a variety of cells and tissues. When a threat to our physical or psychological well-being is detected, the hypothalamus amplifies production of corticotropin-releasing factor (CRH), which induces the pituitary to secrete Adrenocorticotropic Hormone (ACTH). ACTH then instructs the adrenal gland atop each kidney to release cortisol. Together all these changes prepare our bodies to fight or flee and shut down activities that would distract us from self-protection. For instance, cortisol enhances the delivery of fuel to our muscles. At the same time, CRH depresses our appetite for both food and sex and heightens our alertness. Chronic activation of the HPA axis, however, may lay the ground for illness. For each organ system of the body these stress mediators have both short-term adaptive and protective and long-term damaging effects if the stress response is overextended. Examples of adaptive reactions are adjustment of heart rate and blood pressure, increased pressure and increased risk of atherosclerosis, increased risk of type 2 diabetes, cognitive dysfunction, and increased risks of autoimmune and inflammatory disorders.

Two new terms have been used to describe these physiological stress responses: "allostasis," for the adaptive maintenance of stability through change, and "allostatic load," for the wear-and-tear that the body experiences due to over stimulation of allostatic cycles.[5] A person's individual allostatic load represents the biological signature of his or her cumulative psychosocial experience of adversity. Various physiologic parameters (for example, systolic and diastolic blood pressure, waist-hip ratio, serum high-density lipoprotein and total cholesterol, overnight urinary cortisol excretion) have been investigated as measures of allostatic load.

Binary Communication: A communication system with only two response modes such as yes and no, on or off, or 0 and 1 as in informatics. Coma workers may attempt to set up a binary communication link, inviting the patient to use an available movement, like the movement of an eyelid, the mouth, the tongue, a finger or toe, to answer "yes" or "no" to questions. Many movements that coma patients exhibit are not consistent. It takes patience and scrutiny to establish such a communication link. Body processes such as digesting food, fever, and fatigue can interfere with the comatose person's ability to respond. Important questions are best repeated at various times of the day.

City Shadow[6]**:** In Jungian psychology, the shadow or "shadow aspect" is a part of the individual's unconscious mind that consists of the aspects of our personality that we tend to marginalize. Arnold Mindell expanded the shadow concept to whole communities and cities. As communities, we also marginalize aspects of our lives together. Marginalized groups such as psychiatric patients challenge cultural values and norms. They represent the unexplored values and norms of our communities. Coma and other remote states of consciousness also carry a similar shadow aspect that questions cultural norms and values.

Coma: Medically defined as a state in which a patient is not alert and has no awareness, coma can result from structural damage to the brain and from metabolic changes in the body.

Coma and Remote State Directive: Living wills, advance directives, health care directives, and a physician's directive are all documents that a person uses to make known his or her wishes regarding medical treatments such as life-prolonging interventions. Stan Tomandl and Ann Jacob have developed a specific directive for coma care. Please check their Web page at: http://www.comacommunication.com/index.htm.

Contractures: Contractures result in the chronic loss of joint motion due to structural changes in non-bony tissue. These non-bony tissues include muscles, ligaments, and tendons. Contractures lead to shortening of muscles in response to continued heightened muscle tone exerted on that muscle or tendon.

Diffuse Axonal Injury (DAI): DAI is one of the most common and devastating types of traumatic brain injury. The damage to the brain occurs over a more widespread area than in focal brain injury. DAI refers to extensive lesions in white matter tracts and is one of the major causes of unconsciousness and persistent vegetative state after head trauma.[7] It occurs in about half of all cases of severe head trauma. The major cause of damage in DAI is the disruption of nerves and the neural processes that allow one nerve to communicate with another.

The outcome is frequently coma, with over 90 percent of patients with severe DAI never regaining consciousness. Those who do wake up often remain significantly impaired. Unlike brain trauma that happens due to direct impact and deformation of the brain, DAI is the result of traumatic shearing forces that occur when the head is rapidly accelerated or decelerated, as may occur in auto accidents, falls, and assaults. It usually results from rotational forces or severe deceleration. Vehicle accidents are the most frequent cause of DAI; it can also occur as the result of child abuse such as in shaken baby syndrome.

Dreaming Up: This is a Process Work concept that refers to the way our conscious and unconscious signals organize those around us to act as if they are figures in our dreams. For example, a clenched fist and the slight shakiness in our voice are reflections of the things we also dream about. These signals are picked up and "go into" other people around us and they begin to act like those dream figures. One example of this is a man who saw himself as never being angry, but those around him saw him as being very angry. Strange things happened to him—one time he was at a restaurant and someone walked up and punched him in the stomach. The puncher was a dream figure he couldn't own. Unowned figures go out into the world and come back to us as a mirror so that perhaps we can reflect on them and learn more about these unacknowledged parts of ourselves.

Edges: When we reach an edge, it is a place where we feel we can't go any further as we are at the temporary limits of our identity. The edge is the boundary between who I am, in my self concept, and who I am not. For example, I think I am a friendly person, and I don't identify with being powerful, and my edge might be to stand up for myself. At an edge, all kinds of edge figures or dream figures show up with their belief systems that tell us we can't do or be our whole selves.

Entropy: Entropy is a concept of thermodynamics that describes the number of ways in which a system may be arranged. It is often also considered to be a measure of "disorder" (the higher the entropy, the higher the disorder). Increases in entropy correspond to more disorderly and irreversible changes in a system. The energy that is expended as waste heat limits the level of order a system can be in.

Individuation: In Jungian psychology, individuation is a process of psychological differentiation, which has as its goal the development of the individual personality. "In general, it is the process by which individual beings are formed and differentiated; in particular, it is the development of the psychological individual as a being distinct from the general, collective psychology."[8]

Locked in Syndrome/Partial Locked in Syndrome: It is defined as a state in which the patient is fully aware but is not able to, or is only partially able to, express themselves or communicate with their environment. See Bibliography for book and film about locked in syndrome.

Meta Communication: The ability to self-reflect on what you are experiencing. In other traditions, the meta communicator is the witness, the one who can notice and comment on a state while being in the middle of the experience.

Minimally Conscious State: It is a state in which the patient shows some minimal signs of being aware of his or her environment. This condition is distinct from coma or the vegetative state. In minimally conscious states, patients exhibit deliberate behavior. The behavior needs to be consistent enough for clinicians to be able to distinguish it from entirely unconscious, reflexive responses.

Non-locality: The concept from quantum physics that says any personal phenomena or experience is not just personal but is also tied to some larger collective field of experience. Non-locality deals with the interconnectedness of people, objects, and experiences that we ordinarily assume to be separate.

Partial Seizures: These seizures happen when the abnormally excited electrical signals in the brain (seizure) are limited to a specific area of one cerebral hemisphere (side of the brain). Partial seizures are subdivided into simple partial seizures (in which consciousness is retained) and complex partial seizures (in which consciousness is impaired or lost). Partial seizures may spread to cause a generalized or grand mal seizure. Partial seizures are the most common type of seizure experienced by people with epilepsy. Virtually any movement, sensory, or emotional symptom can occur as part of a partial seizure, including complex visual or auditory hallucinations.

Percutaneous Endoscopic Gastrostomy (PEG) Tube: This is the most common type of gastric feeding tube. It is placed endoscopically: the patient is sedated, and an endoscope is passed through the mouth and esophagus into the stomach. The position of the endoscope can be visualized on the outside of the patient's abdomen because it contains a powerful light source. A needle is inserted through the abdomen, visualized within the stomach by the endoscope, and a suture passed through the needle is grasped by the endoscope and pulled up through the esophagus. The suture is then tied to the external end of the PEG tube and pulled back down through the esophagus, stomach, and out through the abdominal wall. The tube is kept within the stomach either by a balloon on its tip (which can be deflated) or by a retention dome, which is wider than the tract of the tube.

Persistent Vegetative State: From a medical viewpoint, it is a state in which the patient is alert but has no awareness. Features that distinguish the vegetative state from other syndromes of lesser brain damage, such as the minimally conscious state, are the absence of sustained visual pursuit (visual tracking) and visual fixation. The eyes do not follow objects or people, nor do they fixate on these objects or people. Persistent vegetative states are generally considered to be **permanent** after three to six months in patients with brain injuries due to lack of oxygen and after one year in patients with traumatic brain injuries.[9]

Process Wisdom/Process Mind/Quantum Mind/BIG YOU: Arnold Mindell uses different terms to describe the organizing power behind your dreaming mind. In his seminal book *Quantum Mind*,[10] he describes the shamanistic, psychological, physical, and mathematical roots of an intelligence that seeks to know itself through a diversity of experiences. Inner and outer diversity, the separation we experience in consensus reality, are both aspects of an organizing principle that guides us toward greater awareness. BIG YOU is the term for the individual thread that connects all our parts, sums up who we are, and gives our life its unique direction. Process wisdom is our active participation in the awareness process. If we use an analogy from the realm of music, your little you is the individual notes of a harmonic sequence, the BIG YOU is the harmony or melodic phrase that gives the notes and parts meaning, and the Process Mind is the creative intelligence behind all music, melodies, and rhythms. It is the intelligence behind your phrasing, timbre, and articulation in the expression of music. Process Mind is the intelligence behind the entangled universe.

Role: Role is a term used in the field of sociology that is frequently used in Process Work. Roles refer to the impersonal behavior patterns that emerge in groups. Roles are often shared by many individuals in a group. Roles are also often internalized and play a part in our individual psychology. Examples of roles are the victim, the smart one, the healthy one, the one in coma, the healer. **Ghost Roles** are hidden roles that are present in a group but not directly spoken for and whose effects are nonetheless felt in the group atmosphere and can be seen in the behavior of group members who react to the Ghost Role. Ghost Roles are referred to or spoken about in conversation. They come up as "gossip" because the group is against the Ghost Role's particular viewpoint or behavior. Bringing awareness to the Ghost Role allows the group to make more conscious decisions and is often felt as relieving.

Sense of Coherence: It is a theoretical construct developed by Aaron Antonovsky[11] that describes our ability to see our lives as manageable, predictable, and meaningful. This personal characteristic has shown to correlate with strong resilience and good health and well being despite internal and/or external challenges.

Spasticity: Spasticity is a disorder of the central nervous system (CNS) in which certain muscles continually receive a message to tighten and contract. Due to brain injury, nerves that regulate muscle tone permanently and continually "overfire" these commands to tighten and contract. This causes stiffness or tightness of the muscles and interferes with gait, movement, and sometimes speech.

Spontaneous Pneumothorax/Collapse of the Lung: A sudden collection of air or gas in the chest causes the lungs to collapse without serious injury. Spontaneous Pneumothrax is caused by a sudden rupture of a bleb or cyst in the lungs.

Synchronicity: Jung defines synchronicity as meaningful coincidences, that is, there is a meaningful connection between two apparently unrelated events.

For example, I am thinking of my sister nonstop and she calls. On a causal level these two things are unrelated, my thinking did not make her call, yet there is a connection on some other level.

Teleological: This philosophical school of thought holds that all things are designed for or directed toward a final result, that there is an inherent purpose or final cause for all that exists, and that order in the universe is not random.

Tracheotomy and Tracheostomy: These are surgical procedures on the neck to open a direct airway through an incision in the the windpipe. People with brain injuries often have an impaired swallowing reflex that can cause dangerous aspiration of food and gastric secretions. Tracheotomy tubes protect patients from breathing in food and gastric secretions.

Wakefulness: Physiologically, wakefulness is based on the intact function of the ascending reticular formation or Ascending Reticular Activating System or ARAS, a set of interconnected nuclei (clusters of neurons) that are located throughout the brain stem which keep us alert. The ascending reticular formation is also called the Reticular Activating System and is responsible for the sleep-wake cycle, thus mediating various levels of alertness.

Notes

INTRODUCTION

1. See Brain Injury Association of America factsheets at: http://www.biausa.org/factsheets.htm.

2. A.M. Owen, M.R. Coleman, M.H. Davis, M. Boly, S. Laureys, and J.D. Pickard, "Using Functional Magnetic Resonance Imaging to Detect Covert Awareness in the Vegetative State," *Archives of Neurology* 64 (2007):1098–1102.

3. Throughout this book we will use various terms to describe our approach. Process-oriented Psychology is a school of thought that was developed by Arnold Mindell and his colleagues in the 1970s. Its roots are in Jungian analytical psychology, Taoism, Field Theory, and Quantum Physics. The applications of Process-oriented Psychology were later called Process Work. Coma Work is one of its applications in the field of palliative and coma care.

4. E. Martin, *Flexible Bodies: Tracking Immunity in American Culture from the Days of Polio to the Age of AIDS* (Boston: Beacon Press, 1994).

5. http://en.wikipedia.org/wiki/Persistent_vegetative_state -_note-taskforce1.

6. Process-oriented Psychology is the mind-body psychology we base this book on. It refers to a body of theory and practice that encompasses a broad range of psychotherapeutic, personal growth, and group process applications. It is more commonly called Process Work in the United States, the longer name being used in Europe and Asia.

7. Arnold Mindell, *Coma, Key to Awakening: Working with the Dreambody Near Death* (New York & London: Penguin-Arkana, 1994).

8. Amy Mindell, *Coma, a Healing Journey: A Guide for Family, Friends and Helpers* (Portland, OR: Lao Tse Press, 1999).

9. Arnold Mindell is the founder of Process-oriented Psychology and Process–oriented Coma Work. It has its origin in Mindell's observation that night-time dreams both mirrored and were mirrored in his clients' somatic experiences, particularly for physical symptoms. He generalized the term "dreaming" to include any aspect of experience that, while possibly differing from consensus views of reality, was coherent with a person's dreams, fantasies, and somatic experience, as well as the unintentional but meaningful signals that form the background to interpersonal relationships.

10. Amy Mindell, *Coma, a Healing Journey*, 11.

11. W.Y. Evans-Wentz, ed., *Tibetan Book of the Dead: or, The After-Death Experiences on the Bardo Plane*, Lama, trans. Kazi Dawa-Samdup (Oxford, UK: Clarendon Press, 1927).

12. Amy Mindell, *Coma, a Healing Journey*, 19.

13. Arnold Mindell, *Coma, Key to Awakening*, 5. Also see Note 6.

CHAPTER 1

1. A.M. Owen, M.R. Coleman, M. Boly, M.H. Davis, S. Laureys, and J.D. Pickard, "Detecting Awareness in the Vegetative State," *Science* 313, no. 5792 (2006): 1402.

2. D.F. Kelly, and D.P. Becker, "Advances in Management of Neurosurgical Trauma: USA and Canada," *World Journal of Surgery* 25, no. 9 (2001):1179–85.

3. Biographical and medical details have been altered to keep the family's privacy.

4. Amy Mindell, *Coma, a Healing Journey: A Guide for Family Friends and Helpers* (Portland, OR: Lao Tse Press, 1999).

5. See Appendix for details about *anoxic brain injuries*.

6. See Appendix for an explanation of *partial seizures*.

7. See Appendix for an explanation of *locked in syndrome*.

8. See Appendix for an explanation of *binary communication*.

9. Arnold Mindell, *Working on Yourself Alone: Inner Dreambody Work* (Portland, OR: Lao Tse Press, 2002).

10. Even though specialized medical knowledge about brain injuries has grown exponentially since 1996, the chances that someone like Matthias would gain from it are still very slim. Functional brain scans are not accessible to most brain injured patients.

11. S. Rosen, *My Voice Will Go with You: The Teaching Tales of Milton H. Erickson, M.D.* (London, W.W. Norton, 1991), 76.

12. http://www.birf.info/support/survivors/successafter.html.

13. See Appendix for a description of *process wisdom*/mind.

14. Arnold Mindell, *Dreaming While Awake* (Charlottesville, VA: Hampton Roads Publishing, 2000), 35–36.

15. Arnold Mindell, *The Quantum Mind and Healing* (Charlottesville, VA: Hampton Roads Publishing, 2004), 17.

16. See Appendix for an explanation of *meta-communication.*

CHAPTER 2

1. B. Jennett, and F. Plum, "Persistent Vegetative State after Brain Damage: A Syndrome in Search of a Name," *Lancet* 1 (1972): 734–737.

2. The Multi-Society Task Force on PVS, "Medical Aspects of the Persistent Vegetative State—First of Two Parts," *New England Journal of Medicine* 330 (1994):1499–1508.

3. J.T. Giacino, et al., "The Minimally Conscious State. Definition and Diagnostic Criteria," *Neurology* 58 (2002): 349–353.

4. C.T. Onions, ed., *The Shorter Oxford English Dictionary* (Oxford: Clarendon Press, 1962).

5. R.L. Solso, *Cognitive Psychology* (Boston: Allyn & Bacon, 2001).

6. J.B. Posner, C.B. Saper, N.D. Schiff, and F. Plum, *Plum and Posner's Diagnosis of Stupor and Coma* (New York: Oxford University Press, 2007).

7. C. McGinn, "Can We Solve the Mind-Body Problem?" *Mind* 98, no. 891 (1989): 349–66.

8. J. Levine, "Materialism and Qualia: The Explanatory Gap," *Pacific Philosophical Quarterly* 64 (1983): 354–61.

9. See Appendix for a more detailed description of the physiology of mind-body interactions.

10. N. Totton, *The Water in the Glass: Body and Mind in Psychoanalysis* (London: Rebus, 1998).

11. Engineers use the concept stress to describe the forces that act on materials and strain them if applied for too long or with too much power.

12. See Appendix entry "Beliefs and Their Role in the Body's Physiology" for an explanation of the physiology of stress.

13. M.E.P. Seligman, T. Rashid, and A.C. Parks, "Positive Psychotherapy," *American Psychologist* 61 (2006): 774–88.

14. A.A. Sheikh, R.G. Kunzendorf, and K.S. Sheikh, "Somatic Consequences of Consciousness," in *The Science of Consciousness: Psychological, Neuropsychological and Clinical Reviews*, ed. M. Velmans (London: Routledge, 1996).

15. K.R. Pelletier, "Between Mind and Body: Stress, Emotions, and Health," in *Mind Body Medicine*, eds. D. Goleman and J. Gurin (New York: Consumer Reports Books, 1993), 19.

16. B. Libet, "Unconscious Cerebral Initiative and the Role of Conscious Will in Voluntary Action," *Behavioral and Brain Sciences* 8 (1985): 529–66.

17. C.S. Soon, M. Brass, H.-J. Heinze, and J.-D. Haynes, "Unconscious Determinants of Free Decisions in the Human Brain," *Nature Neuroscience* 11 (2008): 543–45.

18. W. Pauli, and C.G. Jung, *The Interpretation of Nature and the Psyche* (Princeton, NJ: Pantheon, 1955), 208.

19. The term "consensual" stresses the notion that reality is a cultural concept, not an absolute truth. Arnold Mindell (2000) adds a concept of non-consensus reality that encompasses all spheres of experience that get marginalized (e.g., altered states of consciousness and foggy dreamlike states) in the process of shaping consensus reality by the more dominant parts of society.

20. D. Bohm, *Wholeness and the Implicate Order* (London, Boston: Routledge, 1980).

21. Arnold Mindell, *Quantum Mind: The Edge between Physics and Psychology* (Portland, OR: Lao Tse Press, 2000), 182.

22. K. Wilber, "Waves, Streams, States and Self. Further Considerations for an Integral Theory of Consciousness," *Journal of Consciousness Studies* 7, no. 11–12 (2000): 145–76.

23. Arnold Mindell, *Quantum Mind*, 111.

24. Routine and perfection increase the survival rate of many surgical procedures. Shouldice Hospital outside of Toronto, Canada, has specialized in the surgical repair of hernias. None of their surgeons have completed general surgical training; however, with one year superspecialized training they are the best hernia surgeons in the world.

25. J. Kim, *Mind in a Physical World: An Essay on the Mind-Body Problem and Mental Causation* (Cambridge, MA: MIT Press, 1998).

26. D. Chalmers, "Facing Up to the Problem of Consciousness," *Journal of Consciousness Studies* 2, no.3 (1995): 205.

27. M. Esfeld, "Quantum Holism and the Philosophy of Mind," *Journal of Consciousness Studies* 6, no. 1 (1999): 23–38.

28. S. Hammeroff, "Quantum Vitalism," *Advances: The Journal of Mind-Body Health* 13, no. 4 (1997): 13–22.

29. See Appendix.

30. Arnold Mindell, *Quantum Mind*, 134. See also Note 19.

31. See Note 22.

32. G. Hicks, *One Unknown: A Powerful Account of Survival and One Woman's Inspirational Journey to a New Life* (London: Rodale International, 2007).

CHAPTER 3

1. H. Arendt, "Thinking and Moral Considerations: A Lecture," *Social Research* 38, no. 3(1971): 431.

2. A. Guggenbühl-Craig, "The Archetype of the Invalid and the Limits of Healing," in *The Emptied Soul*, ed. A. Guggenbühl-Craig and J. Hillman (Woodstock, CT: Spring Publications, 1999). For an explanation of the term *archetype*, see Appendix.

3. For an explanation of the term *allopathic*, see Appendix.

4. See "Beliefs Affect Physiologies" in Appendix for further description.

5. V. Frankl, *Man's Search for Meaning* (New York: Washington Square Press, 1984).

6. A. Antonovsky, *Health, Stress and Coping: New Perspectives on Mental and Physical Well-Being* (San Francisco: Jossey-Bass, 1979).

7. For further information see Norman Doidge, *The Brain That Changes Itself: Stories of Personal Triumph from the Frontiers of Brain Science* (New York: James H. Silberman Books, 2007).

8. S. Laureys, M. Boly, and P. Maquet, "Tracking the Recovery of Consciousness from Coma," *Journal of Clinical Investigation* 116 (2006): 1823–25.

9. Ibid., 1824.

10. Ibid., 1823.

11. See Antonovsky, *Health, Stress and Coping*.

12. R.A. Spitz, "Hospitalism: An Inquiry into the Genesis of Psychiatric Conditions in Early Childhood," *Psychoanalytic Study of the Child* 1 (1945): 53–74.

13. J. Bowlby, *Maternal Care and Mental Health* (London: Jason Aronson, 1950).

14. http://www.birf.info/support/survivors/successafter.html.

15. http://www.lifeissues.net/writers/val/val_06_awakenings.html.

16. B. Lown, *The Lost Art of Healing: Practicing Compassion in Medicine* (New York: Ballantine Books, 1999).

17. Ibid., 82.

18. A. Kleinman, *The Illness Narratives: Suffering, Healing, and the Human Condition* (New York: Basic Books, 1988).

19. Arnold Mindell, *Dreambody* (London: Routledge & Kegan, 1984).

20. R. Voelker, "Nocebos Contribute to a Host of Ills," *Journal of the American Medical Association* 275, no. 5 (1996): 345–47.

21. For an explanations of *synchronicity and non-locality*, see Appendix.

22. A. Kleinman, V. Das, and M. Lock, eds., *Social Suffering* (Los Angeles: University of California Press, 1997).

23. J. Andresen, and R.K.C. Forman, "Cognitive Models and Spiritual Maps: Interdisciplinary Exploration of Religious Experience," *Journal of Consciousness Studies* 7, no. 11–12 (2000).

24. See Kleinman et al., *Social Suffering*.

25. For a very good and brief introduction of the Dreambody concept, see Amy Mindell's video at: http://www.aamindell.net/blog/dreambodywork.

26. Arnold Mindell, *The Quantum Mind and Healing* (Charlottesville, VA: Hampton Roads, 2004).

27. See Appendix for an explanation of *process wisdom*.

28. http://www.dailygood.org/more.php?n=3948

29. C. Schnakers, A. Vanhaudenhuyse, J. Giacino, M. Ventura, M. Boly, S. Majerus, G. Moonen, and S. Laureys, "Diagnostic Accuracy of the Vegetative and Minimally Conscious State: Clinical Consensus versus Standardized Neurobehavioral Assessment," *BMC Neurology* 9 (Jul 21, 2009): 35.

30. J. Vikkelsoe, "Beyond Guilt and Innocence: Towards a Process-oriented Criminology." Unpublished doctoral dissertation, Union Graduate School, Cincinnati, OH, 1997, 32.

31. See A. Kleinman, *The Illness Narratives*, and note 25.

CHAPTER 4

1. Arnold Mindell, *Sitting in the Fire* (Portland, OR: Lao Tse Press, 1995), 42.

2. C.G. Jung, M. Meyer-Grass, and L. Jung, eds. *Children's Dreams: Notes from the Seminar Given in 1936–1940* (Princeton: Princeton University Press, 2008), 6.

3. See Appendix for a definition of *dreaming up*.

4. C. Schnakers, A. Vanhaudenhuyse, J. Giacino, M. Ventura, M. Boly, S. Majerus, G. Moonen, and S. Laureys, "Diagnostic Accuracy of the Vegetative and Minimally Conscious State: Clinical Consensus versus Standardized Neurobehavioral Assessment," *BMC Neurology* 9 (Jul 21, 2009): 35.

CHAPTER 5

1. Arnold Mindell, *Quantum Mind and Healing: How to Listen and Respond to Your Body's Symptoms* (Charlottesville, VA: Hampton Roads, 2004), 219.

2. Arnold Mindell, *Earth-Based Psychology: Path Awareness from the Teachings of Don Juan, Richard Feynman, and Lao Tse* (Portland, OR: Lao Tse Press, 2007).

3. See Appendix for a definition of *Process Mind*.

4. See Appendix for a definition of *BIG YOU*.

5. See Mindell, *Earth-Based Psychology*.

6. For a definition of levels of experience, see Chapter 1.

CHAPTER 6

1. Amy Mindell, *Coma, a Healing Journey* (Portland, OR: Lao Tse Press, 1999), 29.

2. Ibid., 275.

CHAPTER 7

1. http://www.cdc.gov/chronicdisease/index.htm.

2. A. Antonovsky, *Health, Stress and Coping; New Perspectives on Mental and Physical Well-Being* (San Francisco: Jossey-Bass, 1979).

3. See Appendix for a definition of *BIG YOU*.

CHAPTER 9

1. L.T. Kohn, J.M. Corrigan, and M.S. Donaldson, eds., *To Err Is Human: Building a Safer Health System* (Washington, DC: National Academy Press, 2000).

2. Arnold Mindell, *Sitting in the Fire* (Portland, OR: Lao Tse Press, 1995).

3. P. Morin. "Rank and Health: A Conceptual Discussion of Subjective Health and Psychological Perceptions of Social Status," *Psychotherapy and Politics International*, Vol 4 (1) (2006), 42–54.

4. S. Griffin, *What Her Body Thought: A Journey into the Shadows* (New York: Harper Collins, 1999), 223.

5. G.A. Kaplan, "Where Do Shared Pathways Lead?" *Psychosomatic Medicine* 57(1995): 208–12.

6. Many people feel constraint if they are perceived in single rigid roles (e.g., as a father). We have many parts and roles and want to be appreciated for all of them. See also Chapter 4.

7. Negative expectations can be transmitted through health professionals' current health beliefs. They can have a great impact on patients' outcomes and chances for recovery (also called nocebo effect). See also Chapter 3.

8. T.S. Kuhn, *The Structure of Scientific Revolutions* (Chicago and London: University of Chicago Press, 1996).

CHAPTER 10

1. http://www.cdc.gov/ncipc/tbi/TBI.htm.

2. http://www.cdc.gov/ncipc/Spotlight/BIAM.htm.

3. Especially if the injury was war related or due to violence.

4. J. Stieglitz, and L.J. Bilmes, *The Three Trillion Dollar War: The True Cost of the Iraq Conflict* (New York. W.W. Norton, 2008).

5. http://discovermagazine.com/2007/mar/dead-men-walking/article_view?b_start:int=1&-C=

6. Institute of Medicine, *Evaluating the HRSA Traumatic Brain Injury Program* (Washington, DC: The National Academy Press, 2006).

7. J.B. Taylor, *My Stroke of Insight: A Brain Scientists Personal Journey* (New York: Viking Penguin, 2008).

CHAPTER 11

1. P. Kapleau, *The Wheel of Life and Death: A Practical and Spiritual Guide* (New York: Doubleday, 1990): 23.

2. J. Garrison, "Rushing Heaven's Door: Assisted Suicide—Do We Really Know What We Want?" *Health* (NY) 11, no. 4 (May-Jun 1997):123–24, 126, 128–30. In this article, Jayne Garrison reports that sociologists at the Mayo

Clinic found that because of aging and illness, people frequently change their mind about what constitutes a "tolerable" life.

3. "Doctors Missing Consciousness in Vegetative Patients." http://www. newscientist.com/article/dn17493-doctors-missing-consciousness-in-vegetative-patients.html?DCMP=NLC-nletter&nsref=dn17493.

4. http://en.wikipedia.org/wiki/Rom_Houben.

5. Sometimes the journey takes another path at life.

6. Arnold Mindell, *City Shadow: Psychological Interventions in Psychiatry* (New York: Routledge, 1988). See Appendix for an explanation of the *city shadow* concept.

APPENDIX

1. Arnold Mindell, *The Dreammaker's Apprentice* (Charlottesville, VA: Hampton Roads, 2001), 151

2. J.W. Kalat, *Biological Psychology* (Belmont, CA: Wadsworth/Thomson Learning, 2001).

3. R. Ader, and N. Cohen, "Behaviorally Conditioned Immunosupression," *Psychosomatic Medicine* 37(1975): 333–40.

4. C. Hertzman, "The Biological Embedding of Early Experience and Its Effects on Health in Adulthood," *Annals of the New York Academy of Sciences* 896 (1999):85–95.

5. B.S. McEwen, and T. Seeman, "Protective and Damaging Effects of Mediators of Stress. Elaborating and Testing the Concepts of Allostasis and Allostatic Load," *Annals of the New York Academy of Sciences* 896 (1999): 30–47.

6. Arnold Mindell, *City Shadow: Psychological Interventions in Psychiatry* (New York: Routledge, 1988).

7. J. Wasserman and R.A. Koenigsberg, "Diffuse Axonal Injury," http://emedicine.medscape.com/article/339912-overview.

8. C.G. Jung. *Psychological Types*, vol. 6, *Collected Works of C.G. Jung* (Princeton: Princeton University Press, 1976), par. 757.

9. The Multi-Society Task Force on PVS, "Medical Aspects of the Persistent Vegetative State," *The New England Journal of Medicine* 330 (1994): 1499–1508.

10. Arnold Mindell, *Quantum Mind* (Portland, OR: Lao Tse Press, 2000).

11. A. Antonovsky, *Health, Stress, and Coping: New Perspectives on Mental and Physical Well-Being* (San Francisco: Jossey-Bass, 1979).

Annotated Bibliography and Coma Work Resources

BIBLIOGRAPHY

Barker, Ellen, ed. *Neuroscience Nursing: A Spectrum of Care.* St. Louis: Mosby Elsevier, 2008.
> Comprehensive nursing textbook that encompasses all neurological disorders. It includes a chapter on neurotrauma and rehabilitation.

Bauby, Jean-Dominique. *The Diving Bell and the Butterfly.* New York: Alfred A. Knopf, 1997.
> Written by a man with locked in syndrome, he provides insight into inner states and communication. Also a great film by the same title.

Beauregard, Mario, and Denise O'Leary. *The Spiritual Brain.* New York: Harper Collins, 2007.
> Based on his study of Carmelite nuns, Beauregard unfolds his ideas about mind over matter and the spiritual experience.

Blackmore, Susan. *Conversations on Consciousness.* New York: Oxford University Press. 2006.
> Susan Blackmore poses intriguing questions to some of the top thinkers in philosophy and brain studies. A good introduction to the fundamental ideas behind the study of consciousness.

Blakely, Mary Kay. *Wake Me When It's Over: A Journey to the Edge and Back.* New York: Times Books, 1989.
> It is a first-person account from inside a diabetic coma. The author "is more lucid in coma than most of us are when wide awake."

Bolte Taylor, Jill. *My Stroke of Insight: A Brain Scientist's Personal Journey.* London: Hodder and Stoughton, 2008.
  A brain scientist describes her personal inner experiences during her stroke.

Boyle, Brian. *Iron Heart: The True Story of How I Came Back from the Dead.* New York: Skyhorse Publishing, 2009.
  Iron Heart is the first-person account of Brian's ordeal and miraculous comeback following the car accident that left him in a coma. He had to learn to talk, then walk, then at last run, and eventually, even to swim. With the dream of competing in the Hawaii Ironman triathlon spurring him on, he defied all medical odds, and three-and-a-half years after the crash, he crossed the finish line in Kona, Hawaii. This is his journey from coma to Kona.

Groves, Richard, and Henriette Anne Klauser. *The American Book of Living and Dying.* New York: Random House, 2009.
  This book is a unique combination of traditional wisdom and modern quantitative and qualitative research around living near death.

Halligan, Peter W., and Derick T. Wade, eds. *The Effectiveness of Rehabilitation for Cognitive Deficits.* Oxford, New York: Oxford University Press, 2005.
  This book covers the treatment of cognitive deficits after brain damage. It doesn't include cognitive rehabilitation of unresponsive patients.

Harrington, Anne. *The Cure Within: A History of Mind-Body Medicine.* New York: W.W. Norton, 2008.
  This book is a very good and comprehensive introduction to the cultural history of mind-body medicine.

Hicks, Gill. *One Unknown: A Powerful Account of Survival and One Woman's Inspirational Journey to a New Life.* London: Rodale International, 2007.
  Gill survived the London Underground bomb attack of 2005 and describes how although she was moving in and out of consciousness and was unable to communicate verbally with her rescuers, she held on to the hand of one of them and could feel him willing her to live and, as she puts it, "sharing some of his life force with her." Later someone else noticed her eyes flickering and used blinking as a way to spell out her name, and she describes her relief at knowing that now they would be able to contact her husband Joe and that helped her to hold on and keep living.

Johanson, Ruthann Knechel. *Listening in the Silence, Seeing in the Dark: Reconstructing Life after Brain Injury.* Berkeley: University of California Press, 2002.
  Author tells the story of her 15-year-old son Erik's recovery from traumatic brain injury after a car accident.

Lawrence, Madelaine. *In a World of Their Own: Experiencing Unconsciousness.* Westport, CT: Praeger Publishers, 1997.
  A nursing instructor researches 100 patients' comatose experiences.

Leon-Carrion, Jose, Klaus R.H. Von Wild, and George A. Zitnay. *Brain Injury Treatment: Theories and Practices.* London, New York: Taylor & Francis, 2006.

A comprehensive medical textbook covering every aspect of neuro-rehabilitation after traumatic brain injury. It promotes/advocates an interdisciplinary holistic program using a team of brain damage specialists (a neuropsychologist, speech therapist, neurologist, psychiatrist, physical therapist, etc.). It includes a chapter on the role of complementary medicine and the role of the family in the rehabilitation process of comatose and brain injured patients. This book is helpful for understanding the complex and difficult treatment processes necessary for optimal medical recovery after brain injury.

Levin, Harvey S., Arthur L. Benton, J. Paul Muizelaar, and Howard M. Eisenberg, eds. *Catastrophic Brain Injury.* Oxford, UK and New York: Oxford University Press, 1996.

This book covers similar ground to the others mentioned above. There are chapters on the pathological features of vegetative states, dealing with the family, research, and moral and ethical issues. This book is written in a clinical style, citing various clinical research, and includes chapters on assessment using brain scanning and other advanced technologies, on pharmacology, and on other more technical aspects of this work. The target audience is professionals. The chapter on families is about getting families to accept the medical assessment and move out of denial.

Le Winn, Edward B. *Coma Arousal: The Family as a Team.* New York: Doubleday, 1985.

We include this book even though it is more than 20 years old as it is a classic, and there are so few other books that deal with different kinds of stimulation in coma. *Coma Arousal* did important groundwork using theory, case studies, and research, to show that stimulation can make a significant difference in recovery rates.

Machado, Calixto, and Alan Shewmon, eds. *Brain Death and Disorders of Consciousness. Advances in Experimental Medicine and Biology,* vol 550. New York: Kluwer Academics/Plenum Publishers, 2004.

This is a collection of papers from an international symposium on coma and death. These proceedings from the conference represent the controversy around coma, persistent vegetative states, and brain death. They critically discuss the conceptual basis of brain death and the philosophical foundations of current mainstream medical thinking about consciousness. This book is written for specialists and health professionals and represents a marginalized voice within the medical community.

Mason, Michael Paul. *Head Cases: Stories of Brain Injury and Its Aftermath.* New York: Farrar, Straus, & Giroux, 2008.

Mason is a brain injury case manager. His stories are powerfully written and captivating. They portray the broad range of people's experiences after brain injury.

Mindell, Amy. *Coma, a Healing Journey: A Guide for Family, Friends, and Helpers.* Portland, OR: Lao Tse Press, 1998.

A practical guide to nonintrusive treatment of patients in altered states of consciousness, especially for people with traumatic brain injury. It covers the basic Coma Work skills and includes very helpful illustrations of the hands-on work.

Amy Mindell presents the pioneering work that she and her husband Arnold Mindell have done in the challenging area of coma care. Mindell shows us that patients who seem to be lost in remote vegetative states in fact give subtle communicative signals. These signals offer the perceptive therapist a channel through which he or she can communicate with the patient and using sensitive communication techniques, understand their experience. Mindell demonstrates how enormously valuable it is to the person in coma when the caretaker connects with the patient's inner experience instead of trying to be a neutral observer or attempting to bring them back to consciousness. Her main theme and concern is that people in all states of consciousness go through potentially meaningful inner experiences. In contrast to modern medical philosophy, she postulates that the potential for awareness still exists as long as the heart is beating.

———. *Metaskills: The Spiritual art of Therapy.* Portland, OR: Lao Tse Press. 1994/2001.

In this book, Amy Mindell describes the deep feeling attitudes for living and interacting with those in all states of consciousness, for instance, curiosity, compassion, and courage.

Mindell, Arnold (forthcoming). *ProcessMind: the Mind of God in Personal Life and in the World's Future.* October 2010 by Quest Books.

———. *City Shadows: Psychological Interventions in Psychiatry.* Portland, OR: Lao Tse Press, 1988/2009.

Mindell includes detailed descriptions of Process Work with people in extreme states. Book pertains to people with dementia and at end of life who could end up in mental hospitals.

———. *Earth-Based Psychology: Path Awareness from the Teachings of Don Juan, Richard Feynman, and Lao Tse.* Portland, OR: Lao Tse Press, 2007.

Drawing from physics, aboriginal beliefs, and shamanism, this book presents new ways of determining the best direction through inner turmoil, relationship trouble, team and community issues, body symptoms, and world issues.

———. *Coma, Key to Awakening: Working with the Dreambody Near Death.* Portland, OR: Lao Tse Press, 1994/2007. (Republished as *Coma: The Dreambody Near Death.*)

This groundbreaking work with people in comas offers new directions in psychotherapy and in the study of people in near-death states.

————. *The Quantum Mind and Healing. How to Listen and Respond to Your Body's Symptoms.* Charlottesville, VA: Hampton Roads, 2004.
Mindell explains how you can access your body's own intelligence and self-healing abilities. Embracing both conventional and alternative medicine, he shows that to truly heal you need both medicine and your own natural wisdom.

————. *The Dreambody in Relationships.* Portland, OR: Lao Tse Press, 2002.
Getting along very well with family, friends, staff, and clients as they emerge from altered consciousness is vital and this volume is life giving.

————. *Working on Yourself Alone: Inner Dreambody Work.* Portland, OR: LaoTse Press, 2002.
Inner work meditation insights and techniques to help learn more about our own inner processes and those of clients and patients.

————. *Sitting in the Fire. Large Group Transformation Using Conflict and Diversity.* Portland, OR: Lao Tse Press, 1995.
In this book, Arnold Mindell shows how attention to power, rank, revenge, and abuse helps build lively and sustainable communities. This book helps understand the power dynamics in care teams and between health professionals and families.

Nader, Robert Shabahangi, and Bogna Szymkiewicz. *Deeper into the Soul: Beyond Dementia and Alzheimer's Toward Forgetfulness Care.* San Francisco: Elders Academy Press, 2008.
The slim volume is a practical guide for people who work and live with relatives or facility residents with dementia. The authors offer ideas and tips for dealing with symptoms, such as aggression and wandering, through conversations between four cartoon figures: a sage, a residential care trainee, a psychologist a social worker, and a physician-researcher, each of whom sees forgetfulness from a different viewpoint.

Posner, Jerome B., Clifford B. Saper, Nicholas D. Schiff, and Fred Plum, eds. *Plum and Posner's Diagnosis of Stupor and Coma,* 4th ed. Oxford, UK and New York: Oxford University Press, 2007.
Seminal medical textbook and cornerstone of medical treatment for comatose patients in virtually every hospital in the United States and Europe. It was originally written in 1952 to differentiate situations that required neurosurgical intervention from those that required medical treatment. It includes the definitions, pathophysiology, and symptoms of coma, and details of the examination, differential diagnosis, and management of the unconscious patient. The current edition discusses the latest scientific discoveries from brain imaging findings that describe islands of consciousness in patients with persistent vegetative states. It also includes a discussion of the ethics of clinical decision making that recommends improving communication with family members. However, it is written for medical professionals from a materialistic standpoint and largely marginalizes the patients' and families' voices.

Reiss, Gary. *Vital Loving: A Guide Book for Couples and Families.* Changing Worlds, 2004.

See Chapter 7: "Family Therapy with Families of Coma Patients."

Richards, Tom. *Eldership: A Celebration,* 2006. http://www.lulu.com/sentientcare.

Tom Richards demonstrates the use of sentient caring skills to encourage eldership in seniors.

Senelick, Richard, MD, and Karla Dougherty. *Living with Brain Injury: A Guide for Families.* Birmingham, AL: Healthsouth Press, 2001.

This book is an introduction to brain functioning and the symptoms and treatment that is standard procedure for brain injuries. It gives a lot of useful information about the different symptoms that go with different levels of brain injury and the diagnostic and treatment routines for these symptoms.

Sullivan, Cheryle. *Brain Injury Survival Kit.* New York: Demos Medical Publishing, 2008.

This book is an all-in-one resource for people with traumatic brain injury and their families. Based on her own experience, Dr. Sullivan provides concrete suggestions and resources.

Tomandl, Stan. *Coma and Remote State Directive,* 1991. http://www.lulu.com/sentientcare.

This Web site offers a living will for those concerned with communication and decision making during states of confusion, delirium, stupor, coma, catatonia, advanced dementia, and other so-called remote states of consciousness.

———. *Coma Work and Palliative Care: An Introductory Skills Manual for Supporting People Living in Coma Near Death.* 1991. http://www.lulu.com/sentientcare.

A bedside manual that contains detailed techniques for working with people in metabolic coma, altered consciousness, and advance dementia near death.

Tomandl, Stan, and Tom Richards. *An Alzheimer's Surprise Party: New Sentient Communication Skills and Insights for Understanding and Relating to People with Dementia,* 2006. http://www.lulu.com/sentientcare.

Dr. Arnold Mindell strongly recommends this as an original method for understanding and dealing with Alzheimer's and dementia.

Winslade, William J. *Confronting Traumatic Brain Injury: Devastation, Hope, and Healing.* New Haven: Yale University Press, 1998.

This book offers an excellent overview of the field of Coma Work and specifically traumatic brain injury. It briefly covers the anatomy and physiology of the brain and what happens in brain injury, and discusses cutting-edge research, for example, with hyperbaric therapy and head injuries. It also says what rehabilitation consists of, and touches briefly on ethics around this work.

COMA WORK RESOURCES

American Academy for the Certification of Brain Injury Specialists: http:// www.aacbis.net.

> The mission of the Academy of Certified Brain Injury Specialists (ACBIS) is to improve the quality of care given to individuals with brain injury through the education and training of those who work in brain injury services. To that end, ACBIS offers a voluntary national certification program that establishes best practices for the training of individuals working with this population. Because of the wide variety of unique skills and knowledge required of those who treat persons with brain injury, certification is designed to address specific training issues in brain injury services and to complement other existing credentials.

Brain Injury Association of America (BIAA). 1608 Spring Hill Road, Suite 110, Vienna, VA 22182. Phone: (703) 761-0750. Toll-free: (800) 444-6443. Fax: (703) 761-0755. http://www.biausa.org.

> BIAA provides information, education, and support to individuals, families, and professionals whose lives are affected by brain injury. It also publishes the National Directory of Brain Injury Rehabilitation Services.

Brain Injury Recovery Kit (BIRK). BIRK is currently the only do-it-yourself rehabilitation kit for survivors and their caretakers. It offers a practical "Keys to Recovery" system that addresses cognitive impairments common to survivors. Visit http://www.daytimer.com/birk or http://www.10in10project.org.

The Centers for Disease Control and Prevention, National Center for Injury Prevention and Control; Traumatic Brain Injury information page: http://. www.cdc.gov/ncipc/tbi/TBI.htm.

Defense and Veterans Brain Injury Center (DVBIC). DVBIC is a multisite medical care, clinical research, and education center funded through the Department of Defense. You can sign up for the DVBIC newsletter at http://www.dvbic.org.

Epilepsy Foundation: http://www.epilepsyfoundation.org.

National Association of State Head Injury Administrators (NASHIA). http:// www.nashia.org.

> NASHIA acts as point of contact for caretakers, professionals, or other state employees seeking information about availability of services, grants, or programs specific to their state.

National Institute of Neurological Disorders and Stroke (NINDS). National Institutes of Health, The Neurological Institute, P.O. Box 5801. Bethesda, MD 20824. http://www.ninds.nih.gov.

NeuroRehabilitation: An Interdisciplinary Journal. http://www.iospress.nl.

New Scientist Topic Guides: The Human Brain. http://www.newscientist.com/topic/brain.

North American Brain Injury Society (NABIS). http://www.nabis.org.
    NABIS is comprised of brain injury professionals. They disseminate effective, science-based treatment, and education.
Traumatic Brain Injury.com. Suite 1705, Two Penn Center Plaza, Philadelphia, PA 19102–1865. http://www.traumaticbraininjury.com.

Index

About the Authors

PIERRE MORIN, MD, PhD is co-president of the International Association of Process-oriented Psychology (IAPOP), faculty member at the Process Work Institute of Portland, and teaches Process oriented Psychology worldwide. He was the assistant clinical director of Switzerland's leading rehabilitation clinic for brain injuries for five years. He currently works in Portland, Oregon, as a clinical director in an outpatient mental health program and in private practice. Dr. Morin has written several articles on mind-body medicine and community health.

GARY REISS, LCSW, PhD is in private practice in Eugene and Portland, Oregon, as a therapist. He is a senior faculty member of the Process Work Institute of Portland and teaches Process-oriented Psychology worldwide. He has worked with coma and head injury recovery patients in many different countries and is one of the developers of Process-oriented family therapy. He is the director of the Process Work Institute Rivers Way student clinic. He has written *Changing Ourselves, Changing the World*; *Vital Loving*; *Angry Men, Angry Women, Angry World*; and *Beyond War and Peace in the Arab Israeli Conflict*.